A Pillar of

Mark Edgar

chipmunkapublishing
the mental health publisher

Mark Edgar

Published by
Chipmunkapublishing
PO Box 6872
Brentwood
Essex CM13 1ZT
United Kingdom

http://www.chipmunkapublishing.com

Edited by Neal Swami

Cover design Beka Smith

Chipmunkapublishing gratefully acknowledge the support of Arts Council England.

Author Biography

Mark Edgar was born in Surrey in 1969. Educated as a chorister at Kings College Cambridge and a music scholar at Lancing College, he returned to Cambridge in 1988 as a choral exhibitioner at Selwyn College where he read history. It was whilst at Cambridge, aged 20, that mental illness first struck. Despite the illness he managed to graduate with a 2.1 in 1991.

Following many years of illness and living on benefits he managed to return to Cambridge for a third time in 1999 to undertake a Post Graduate Certificate in Education and was awarded Qualified Teacher Status in August 2000. Unable to find a teaching job he worked as a part time Learning Support Assistant at South Kent College on a specialist course aimed at getting people with long term mental health difficulties back into education.

Following on from occasional work for Mind since 1995, in 2002 he almost fell into working in mental health full time, initially with Kent Social Services and then Rethink. A second stint with Social Services followed in 2005 before a move to the University of Hertfordshire in September 2007 as their very first Mental Wellbeing Advisor.

Mark started writing in 1997. He won the Rethink Pringles award for art and poetry in 2002 with his poem *The Archbishop's Palace*. Work on *A Pillar of Impotence* began in 2002 and was completed in 2005. He also contributed a chapter to *Voicing Psychotic Experience, a Reconsideration of Recovery and Diversity* which was published in 2009.

Although he rarely sings now he retains an interest in music. He has a passion for American Football having played in Cambridge and coached in Kent, and enjoys watching cricket and rugby. His other great passion in life is cooking foods from all round the world.

Mark Edgar

Special thanks go to the following people who played a significant role in either the writing of the book or in my story:

Jason Pegler and Paul Kirven at Chipmunkapublishing. My readers Jayne Curry, Jody Winter, Jan Munns, and Katie O'Brien. To Beth Hart for the photo that adorns the e book version and her wonderful support throughout the writing period. Beka Smith for the artwork. To my friends in Cambridge, Christopher Kelly, David Smith, and Michael Tilby who never stopped believing I would come back from mental illness. The remarkable Caroline Latham who first gave me the hope that I could recover. Ian Morrison who believed in and supported that recovery. Christine Counsell who allowed me to fulfil my dream of returning to Cambridge. James Padley will always be remembered for making me engage again with the world beyond mental illness. Ruth Chandler and Laura May for their assistance with editing. Heather Murray my long time friend, supporter, and advocate. The final thanks goes to Dr Heather McAlister who finally saw through the fog of my illness, thought outside the box, ignored my notes, and came up with a simple and lasting solution; a psychiatrist of rare ability who sadly left my life all too quickly.

Mark Edgar

For my friends who died too young.

Mark Edgar

Chapter 1

Sleep in Heavenly Peace

Where is she? Why didn't she come? She promised she'd come. Maybe she doesn't care. Maybe she lied. She wouldn't do that. The myriad of thought kept cascading through my head. It hadn't stopped for over a year. It never slowed down and could never be switched off, just an endless stream over which I had no control. Even in the days before, I had never been able think with such clarity and speed. No deliberate effort at thinking had ever matched this. But at least then I could switch off at times, and it usually had a purpose, a direction. At least I had been able to achieve then rather than destroy myself. I just want to sleep!

Between the thoughts came the voice, in alternation with the conscious but uncontrolled. That haunting, echoing voice that showed so little emotion but brought so much pain. She spoke, and through my thought I spoke to her, but she never gave me answers. We spoke for hours, connected yet unconnected. I never knew when she'd speak, but she was always there, a shadow of great joy but intense pain. There was never a day without her, just breaks when she was inert rather than active. Why won't she come? Why won't she go? The thoughts intruded into the conscious again. She promised. Where is she?

The summer was drawing on, August, nearing its end. What had happened to that summer? A few short weeks from the moments that were supposed to have been such a triumph. Education for life, the great culmination of all those years of study. Cambridge was over. The triumph had never come, at least for me, just a continuation of this sense of impending disaster. Summer drew towards its end but what else was ending? Those few short weeks of the summer had meant nothing, no escape. I had always had somewhere to escape to, back to Cambridge but there was no way back this time. In those weeks the sense that I had moved from losing the fight to have the will to live, to actively wanting to die had merely intensified. There was no getting away from it, just an active pursuit of it. It had happened right at the end, just the realisation that it was the only answer to chaos that had become me.

Triumph to disaster, but disaster for whom? It had been anything but a sense of triumph, just another step towards the nothing that awaited me afterwards. There was just a sense of nothing, just more and more pain. Why won't the thinking stop? I want to sleep. I'm going to die. I want to die. More thoughts.

They'd given me some pills. "They'll help you to sleep" they'd said. The little yellow pills, the ones that they had neglected to tell me what they were. That was the simple solution. Take the pills and be better, get the sleep I so desperately craved. But sleep never came, at least not usually until dawn or later. Then the call: "it's 8 o' clock, it's time to get up." There always had to be some air of normality because that was what normal people did. They got up then because it's normal. Day in day out it had been the same through that summer. Two, three, four hours sleep per night. The more tired I got the worse the thinking got; the worse the thinking got the less sleep I got. An endless cycle with no way out. Only death and it would be self induced. That had been an absolute since the end of Cambridge. A tunnel from which there was no deviation, or any intention to escape. I had long since become too tired even to want to fight the idea. I had the plan, to use the car. A simple solution, but I needed the garage, and could not get it until September. I just had to wait and suffer until then.

The car was parked over the road late that summer. The neighbours had offered to keep it off the road. "It's safer over there," they'd said. Parked on the slope by their garage, the reverse hill start to get back on the road. So much was said by such people but it all meant nothing. It sat under the tree collecting a sticky residue as summer moved towards autumn. It always struck me, in a strange way that this seemed to reflect what was happening. Thicker layers as I moved further and further into the swamp. However much I tried to clean it off, it always remained, just as there was no way forward for me. Just an ever deepening sense of drowning, and efforts to help, such as they were, were just too late.

I loved that car. The battered yellow VW with the scratched paintwork at the front, and the cracked indicator light, where I'd crashed into an ambulance. No one was hurt, I was just shaken, and then we all went on our way. We'd all thought it highly amusing to crash into something like that. But that was in the days when things were going so well and we'd had so much fun. Things had moved on so far in little more than a year.

The car was all that was left. The remnants of a legacy long spent, spent trying to stave off the pain. Above all it was mine and no one else's, something no one else could take away. It had been a means of joy, of escape, of travel, a God send. Without it I would have arrived at that point far earlier. Now it was to be the means to another end, to the ultimate escape, my means of life and my means of death. I had chosen very carefully, weighing it up, how to die with the least pain to me, and to cause the least inconvenience to others. I'd often thought how unpleasant it would be to be the train driver you jumped out on, the person in the car you deliberately drove into. It had never crossed my mind that I would be found by someone. The thinking had been both entirely logical and entirely mixed up. There was always a hose pipe in some God forsaken field, but there was too much risk in that. No one should have the chance to stop it. That's why I needed the garage, but I couldn't get it until September to be undisturbed. I'd waited a long time, but the time was coming as the season drew on. It was stuck by a garage but it was still on the road.

That road. We'd lived there since I was nine, but I'd never really lived there. Just resided there in the holidays when there was nowhere else to go. At the end of one summer term, the school friends actually presented me with a rota of places to stay, just to escape. It had covered from July to September, a week here, ten days there. I'd thought it was a joke but they'd meant it. Perhaps I should have taken them up on the offer, but I always had to return there in the end and face the inevitable enmity.

Cambridge had offered greater opportunities, but greater pitfalls. There was the freedom of the car, but there were also the interminably long holidays. In my first year I'd stayed for two weeks of the long vacation on the pretence that I had to catch up on work missed earlier in the year. This was a lie. It was just another chance to escape, if only for a short while. It was never long enough, and always the same on the return. Now there was nowhere left to escape to. Stuck there, alone with my thoughts. Just so very alone.

I sat in the car late that warm August night, secretly whiling away the hours before trying to sleep. Everything had become so secretive, my movements, my thoughts, my actions. Must be quiet, no one must know. These thoughts above all else pervaded my existence. In my place, chain smoking, desperately fighting the thoughts as they came in waves. I listened so quietly to Marley, the music of the oppressed, the mournful sounds of Mclean, in my time. Mustn't wake the neighbours. Where is she? Why didn't she come?

I was due to go away on one of my many trips within a few days, and had a full bottle of the little yellow pills for the trip. Through the disorder a calming clarity began to emerge. Fuck the garage, I have the pills. Surely they'll do the trick. This revelation had never been part of the plan but seemed so helpful as things stood. No need to wait for the garage, just take them and go. The plan was now redundant, but the satisfaction of quicker escape was immense. The end was finally in sight and I was energised to act with great surety. An enormous sense of relief, peace, and satisfaction engulfed me. Are there enough pills? Do I need more?

With Marley finished I emerged very quietly and rummaged through the boot for the remnants of the pain killers I had used some months before. I was convinced that the extra pills would do the trick, even though I had no idea of the toxicity of either. There was no thought of failure after I'd found them, and quietly I locked the boot and the door, in automatic reaction to leaving the car for the night. The thought that that was irrelevant never crossed my mind. I just had a single-minded purpose that blotted out all thoughts, rational or otherwise.

I slowly climbed the steps to the house, and, quietly as possible opened the door, as I was wont to do that late. No one must hear me. Just as quietly and slowly I walked upstairs and collected the bottle of yellow pills. Back in the kitchen I drew a large glass of water and contemplated the pills. Would they taste of anything? Would it be easy? Could I do it? The only thought I didn't have was that maybe I didn't want to take them. I took the pain killers first, bigger but with a slightly sweet taste. That was easy. I opened the second bottle and took a mouthful. Then a mouthful of water and swallowed. There was a chalky texture where each pill had collided with the others in the bottle, the dust of storage. Another mouthful and swallow. Then another, then the last. It had been just so easy. No fear, just a normal function, just like quenching one's thirst on a hot day.

I refilled the glass, and in total darkness moved towards the stairs. Must keep quiet. Mustn't wake anyone. As I climbed the stairs, a flattened palm guided me along the wall, an art well practised that summer. It was slow progress but a great serenity had descended on my mind and it was simply a case of waiting just a few minutes longer. Finally, after a perceived age, I made my destination.

Once in my room, I changed and carefully folded my clothes and placed them on the chair; another ironic gesture. The final thought was that it was, at long last, going to be over. Calm still pervaded my head, a calm I'd not known for so long. It was so easy. I got into bed and lay down to die.

Chapter 2

Balls and Bumps

I emerged unusually early from the gloom of C staircase. It was about two hours earlier than my habitual time for rising during the term, especially now that exams had finished, and we looked forward to the rest of an anticipatedly frantic May Week. It was far too bright to cope with at that time of the morning, and though already warm, I expected another very hot day as we headed for the last day of the Bumps. They had gone wrong the day before, and the dream of Blades was gone, but what a race it had been on that Friday. Part of the targeted trilogy of successes had gone, but the other two still stood.

The lack of sleep and hangover were far from helped by the brightness of the day. My myopia was proving to be a major handicap that day. Having only taken my lenses out an hour or two before, I was confronted by the harsh reality of either being able to see with my glasses and be dazzled by the sun, or go virtually blind into the world that Saturday morning with shades to block out the intensity of the light. In view of the hangover, the time of the morning, and the chronic lack of sleep the night before, the latter appeared to be a much better option. As the next few minutes panned out, short-sightedness was to prove the least of the handicaps on that day.

As I was walking down from the third floor, I was reflecting on the revelries of the previous day. It was a strange coincidence that in all my years in Cambridge, I always ended up on the top floor of the building, in Cripp's, in Old Court, and, years later on my return. I suppose it gave me more time to reflect as I went up and down. Cambridge May Balls seemed such a wonderful institution at the time. Decadence gone crazy, and, at that stage, few, if any of us, realised that the decadence that had been the late 1980s was about to be lost for ever. Balls were a wonderful opportunity to get dressed up, eat, drink, listen, watch, and have a great deal of fun. Everything was free, in a manner of speaking, once the cost of the ticket had been discounted. Fortunately, here the cost was not too extortionate, unlike at some other colleges. At the time, money was not really much of an issue as I had recently come into a small legacy. Anyway, it was inconceivable that we would not go to the Ball, despite the fact that we had to row the next day, the last day of the Bumps. Nothing was really destined to stop a night of great drunkenness, and whatever else that night was to bring. It was the culmination of a year for those who had worked, or were supposed to have worked hard, and above all, liked to play harder.

It had been a great night. Much better than the previous year, when the nervousness that can affect those new to the institution that was Cambridge, was still partly in evidence. Great food, huge amounts to drinks, many friends to see and enjoy the night with. The intention was always to get through without sleep at all, at least until the Survivors photo at around 7 or 8 o' clock. I'd certainly made it through the night, but missed the actual photo. The plan was then to sleep as long as possible until the time when thoughts had to be collected for the impending race later in the afternoon or evening. All in all, the weekend had a great deal of promise, the Ball, the Bumps, Suicide Sunday, and as an accident of fate that year, the Boat Club Dinner on that Sunday evening too. We'd all mused on the error the college's ways by allowing the Dinner to be on that Sunday after a day of such unmitigated drunken carnage. But since it had to happen, we had to do it. It would have been a bad show if we had failed to take this opportunity.

It promised to be a great day for watching rowing; bright, sunny and hot. Probably not so good to be actually racing due to the anticipated heat, but perfect for big crowds down the course. But not at all perfect at that time of the morning, having singularly failed to achieve the sleep part of the plan. Short-sightedness was definitely a better idea at that time, not really a problem knowing Cambridge as well as I did. But this was not the only slightly small cloud of difficulty that day. I had the prospect of having to see my family that day. For reasons that I failed to understand, they wanted to come up to see the Bumps. I never did work out why it was that event rather than one of the many other things that littered Cambridge life for me, that they had chosen to come and see. They had, however, decided to come, and I faced the prospect of returning to the usual life of deception that I lived away from Cambridge. I had no desire for anyone to intrude into this part of life, escape as it was. It had always been selected parts of my life that had pleased them, rather than the parts I liked best. But at least, for once, it was something not musical that had attracted their attention. There was also the thorny prospect of having to go home for those incredibly long holidays I was forced to endure at Cambridge. That morning though, future thoughts were not playing a large part in the equation of today.

The second year had gone so well. I was so much more integrated into our world than I had been. Constantly surrounded by people, and so busy, time had slipped by with much fun and enjoyment. Academically things had worked out extremely well, with some of the tutors predicting the first that I had so coveted since arriving. As far as I was concerned, I'd done enough, and things had gone well in the exams. I had been very aware of the potential for the element of luck. But luck could work both ways. At the very least there was the 2:1, which would do, but I would always regret. Perhaps it was arrogance, or maybe self belief.

I'd continued to sing, although I found that very dull in Cambridge. I'd continued to play American Football for the University, and despite the concussion, and subsequent despair in the Varsity Match, the prospects for the following year, when I was to be President, were looking good. Rugby still continued, and in the summer, after much persuasion from friends, I had finally taken up the noble art of rowing and coxing, much to the feigned disgust of my tutor. But above all, it was the great camaraderie that had made that year so good. To cox a boat, and be that much of a team player was something new to me, much more evident than in so many other sports I'd played. And of course, that inevitably translated into other areas of college life. Whatever one's view of the respective college Boat Clubs, good or bad, it had been a great experience for me. Later that day, that boat would go into action for the last time, as that group of people. The Blades had gone, but the upbeat nature that had emerged that year was still in evidence. One part of the target for the year lost, but still two to go and the signs appeared, at least to me, to be good.

The thorny issue of the holidays was less of a problem than it had been before. At last I was mobile with my own car, and I didn't have too much of a problem financing it. There would be many parties and opportunities to get away during the summer. I didn't really anticipate that what we had in college during the term time, would be that different in the holidays, just a bit less regular, and a bit more spread out in time. Plans were already afoot to go on holiday later in the summer. It would finally be a chance to get away without having to sing. That would be very different to the norm. I was, to all intents and purposes, in a much better position than I'd ever found myself before going into the summer holidays. But there was much to do before that happened, fun to be had, parties, people, and whatever happened to turn up. There was still time before the end of term, and I had every intention of enjoying it. Just a few distractions, like the temporary appearance of the family today.

The other sense within my musing that morning was the hint of guilt, a feeling of self justification for the actions of the previous night. Although only a small feeling at that stage, there was, nevertheless, that thought of having done something terribly wrong, but not really mattering; like having an extra biscuit as a child when told you could only have one. As I walked into the court I was followed by the girl from the night before, the American, the girl from Alabama. She was friend of a close friend, visiting the UK for part of the summer. She'd been brought to the Ball separately by those friends; we'd met, and hit it off. It was just another of those accidents in life, a chance meeting. Nothing had been intended or expected on my part, but as the night drew on, we got closer together, and wound up back in my rooms early that morning. I'd been with her at the time of the Survivors photo, awake and aware, just not available.

As she hardly knew Cambridge, I'd told her hostess that I would bring her back in the morning to Portugal Place, before having to go back to meet the family and prepare for the rowing. It had been the intention for us then to all meet up at some stage later in the day for a few post rowing drinks. So it was that we set out from C staircase for the leisurely stroll back, a trip I was forced to undertake tired, hangover, and with little ability to see.

The court was unusually shambolic as the remnants of the previous night were cleared up, marquees taken down, and the ropes, pegs, and canvasses packed up to move on to the next venue. It was a rare sight to see the hallowed lawns of Old Court in such a state, and the marks on the grass where the tents had been, were clearly visible, lighter in colour than the unmarked areas. The lawns were reserved for the Fellows to walk across, and Ball tickets always seemed to bear the message "By the Kind Permission of the Master and Fellows..." Walking on the grass was a privilege reserved for such occasions as these. As we crossed the Court, I decided to go to the pigeon holes to see if there was any post. It was always the practise of the porters to clear out the post on the day of the Ball, as a means to safeguard any correspondence from any overly exuberant drunk who, in such a state, might cause unnecessary damage or loss. The post was always put back or delivered the next morning so life wasn't interrupted too much.

When we got there, I found a letter from a very unexpected source sitting there waiting for me. The slight pangs of guilt grew a little stronger within me, but were not visible to anyone else. It was just a sense of irony standing there with that letter in my hand, with the American girl standing next to me. It was from Rachel, but was totally unexpected. We'd spoken at length the previous afternoon from the call box up the road. She'd wished me luck in the Bumps, hoped that I enjoyed the Ball, and generally perused the idea of the fun I was having after the exams, and dullness of her present position. The one thing she had not mentioned was that she had written to me, and that the letter was in the post as we spoke. Hence, my feeling of surprise to be there with an unexpected letter from her, with the girl from Alabama by my side. It was always pleasing to receive letters from her, always rather more permanent than phone calls and odd conversations. It had always been difficult with her in one part of the country, and me in another. Despite the irony and sense of guilt, I was very pleased to have heard from her. Rather than wait to open it on my return, I decided to open it and read it as we went towards Portugal Place. Perhaps it suited my rather devious and ironic nature; Rachel and the American in the same space and time frame.

As we walked back in the direction of C staircase, and on to the gate to West Road, I opened this surprise letter. Holding it quite close so I could actually see it, I began to read. "This is bad, really bad" was all that I was able to mumble, as it became rapidly clear that Rachel was gone. None of it made a great deal of sense as it was so unexpected. Just line after line of apologies and intentions, but nothing at all about why. No explanation, just trying to be as nice as possible. Nothing was ever quite the same after that moment.

Another of those ironies that seem to plague life, that sense of guilt I had vaguely been feeling was proved to be completely irrelevant. I briefly mused on the idea that one couldn't really be unfaithful if one had parted ways already, did it therefore matter that I hadn't known? I wasn't angry, just really confused. There had been no inclination that things were different or wrong when we'd spoken the previous afternoon. I couldn't conceive the idea of being able to hide behind this bland, but permanent record of intention. Why hadn't she said anything? The thoughts started to rush at me with alarming rapidity. Why?; what?; how?; where next? This was the start of a process that was to plague me for many years.

At the same time I was trying to get the American back. How much, if anything, she sensed I have no idea. I did, however, feel secure in my thoughts. I'd always taken pride in being able to hide what I truly felt or thought. Many years of practise at being something I was not, kicked into my conscious. As we walked through the streets of Cambridge, she had no idea what she had just witnessed, in either a simple or complex way. It was to be another year before anyone was to realise the severity of the damage that fateful journey had on my mind. As we walked, I was overwhelmed by a desire to be alone. It seemed imperative that I should not display publicly what effect that letter had had on me. After all, no one had seen the contents of the letter, still less understand the impact it had and was to have. We chatted as we walked. Mustn't give anything away. Thoughts forming and repeating on themselves. Oh shit, I've got to meet my parents later. That was the last thing I could handle at the time.

We made it to Portugal Place, and, after the usual banter, I turned for the return journey. At last I could be alone with my feelings and thoughts. The thoughts continued to take over. Above all was this idea of why. None of it made sense. More important was the sense of incredible aloneness. It overwhelmed me, and for the first time I realised that all the norms of reality seemed to have moved in my perception. Everything that I knew and trusted seemed to have shifted out of place. I quickly began to distrust my senses. Why hadn't I felt like this in the past when things had broken down? Why is it different? What the fuck is going on?

Then the reality of the rest of the day began to settle in. You've got to sort yourself out for the Bumps. You've got to pretend for the coming family visit. You've got the Boat Club Dinner, tomorrow's Suicide Sunday. It will be great once you've got that visit out of the way. None of these thoughts, good or bad, changed the feeling of catastrophe. I felt completely lost as I walked slowly back, the shades covering my tired and unseeing eyes, and the feelings that lay hidden away. The shades were to become a recurring theme for many years to come, as I sought desperately to hide away, and avert the physical pain that was to come later.

A couple of hours after getting back to college, my parents arrived. I felt exhausted and not really there. For the first time I used what was to become a moniker for me over the years, "I'm just really tired". I think they sensed that it was far more than that, but like me, it didn't make any sense to them either. My mother was to say afterwards that "it was as if you were a totally different person". She was, of course, right, but since she knew so little of who I was before, it was a comment that had little meaning for me. The right thing to say but for the wrong reason. I really couldn't handle seeing them at all that day, and it began to dawn on me that the long summer of isolation was coming up remarkably quickly. If I can't handle them now for just a few hours, what the fuck are the holidays going to be like? Another shift in the thoughts, but still no move away from what was really going on; just more anticipated problems.

My mind was still being consumed as I arrived with the crew at the river later in the afternoon. I felt completely unable to focus on the task in hand, but was determined to make a good showing in this final race together as a crew. At the start the exhilaration of the action was there, the crowds were loud, and the atmosphere was ecstatic, but it was all dulled within my head. The day was a disaster for the boat, caught by a crew we had bumped on the first day. The usual bullshit of a "touch of the May Balls," "well rowed," and "bad luck." There was probably a great deal of truth in what was said: it was clearly not such a good idea to row a serious race when we'd been up all night drinking. But that all meant nothing to me; in my head and my thinking, it was me that had fucked up by not being focused on what I was supposed to be thinking about. That thought was to become deeply entrenched in my mind. I was always to believe that it was my fault, and no logical argument could change that.

We spent the rest of the day as we always did in May Week, drinking heavily, recounting the stories of the day, and generally celebrating. We knew what tomorrow would bring as we would open the batting with the home brewed stout party at 9 o' clock, followed by endless Pimm's at various garden parties, then the Dinner. It was, after all, Suicide Sunday. I tried to forget as we drank and looked forward, but the sense of isolation continued. I felt the need to hide it from the others, and never did find out if anyone was sober enough to have noticed. Two parts of the target were now gone for ever. But it was Rachel who mattered above all else. She was gone, and somehow I had to find out what to do next. I had no idea where I was going to find the answer to all of this. If there was an answer.

The thoughts just continued as I went to bed. Little sleep was achieved that night either, but for a very different reason. Life was very hazy. I felt lost in a totally alien place, and I had absolutely no idea where to turn, or what to do to get out. My world, as I perceived it, had changed irrevocably that day. Little of what was around me was clear after that day. The illness started that day.

Chapter 3

The Cock Crowed Thrice

Suicide Sunday was the usual grand affair, decadence personified. Self-indulgent over excess from early in the morning. After the home brewed stout party we all adjourned to the rather beautiful college gardens, which always looked decidedly shabby within hours of us starting, let alone by the time we'd finished. Weekends in the summer were usually punctuated by at least one garden party a week. Grand invitations were sent out with some regularity "requesting the pleasure of your company" at a certain time in the gardens. One was required to bring a prescribed quantity of Pimm's, vodka, sparkling wine, or some other concoction for the day's drinking. Dress was usually blazers, with members of the various drinking societies required by some form of statute, or penalty, to wear a particular tie. Industrial size food serving trays were procured from the kitchens, with the group or individuals taking responsibility for returning these at the close of proceedings. Some form of cocktail was then made, top ups coming as more people arrived. Plastic cups were issued, and one then just proceeded to help one's self until the alcohol ran out, or in many cases, as long as one could still stand. Suicide Sunday was the embodiment of the garden party ethos that pervaded Cambridge in the summer term, and to an extent, the long vacation as well. It was the civilised thing to do when the summer sun came in occasional abundance.

What set Suicide Sunday apart from all other days, was that a whole series of parties took place right across the university, throughout the day, with many following on in the same place as the day progressed. We had five such parties taking place that day, following on from one another, in the college gardens. The people running them changed but the drinkers didn't. It just meant going off every couple of hours to get more alcohol, of the required denomination. In the days of restricted selling of alcohol, and being a Sunday, it was almost impossible to get anything before midday, and all shops tended to sell out of Pimm's by about one o' clock at the latest. It always paid to think ahead and stock up beforehand. Essential in fact since proceedings started at nine o clock, although the stout had been brewing since the beginning of term. As expected, it tasted foul but it was "the taking part that counts". I never did work out if it was a good or bad way to start the day.

Party followed party, but we broke for a brief siesta at some point in the afternoon. Having finished the afternoon session, I struggled into Black Tie in preparation for the Boat Club Dinner. It was to be the first time in a number of years that the Boat Club was allowed to dine actually in college, punishment for the sins of our forefathers no doubt. In anticipation of drunken difficulties later, we'd been required by the college to organise a post dinner event outside of Old Court, over the road. This was to be, inevitably, a cocktail party. Dinner went off extremely well, although the stroke of my boat never made it past the first course. I had a vague recollection of dancing on a table precariously close to the portrait of the founder of the college, but no damage was done. We went to the cocktail party, and finally to the pub until closing time, just to round off the day.

It proved to be a monumental day, even by the hallowed standards of the Boat Club. I'm sure the college regretted that the Hall had been double booked on the Saturday so the Dinner had to take place on Suicide Sunday, but little or no lasting damage was done. Everyone enjoyed what they could remember of the day, despite the hangovers, with many stories to be told for the future. I remembered the day rather better than most. Throughout the day, despite the effects of the Pimm's, my mind was in another place. I tried hard to work out what to do, yet at the same time, sought to escape the situation that still made no sense. Try as I might, I completely failed to get away from how I felt about the events of the previous morning. Why do I feel like this? Why is it different? How do I deal with this? I was completely lost in those thoughts. I was strangely oblivious to that around me, but at the same time profoundly aware of that which was going on around me. The day was great but it was as if I was living it from behind a mask of my own invention; I was there but not there. Everything had taken on a peculiar falseness to it, something I had never experienced before. I felt completely out of my depth, participating yet watching from a great distance. I had fond memories after the day, but they were tainted by this detachment. I was trying to tell myself that the feelings would pass in time, yet something told me immediately that they would not. This was far from a normal, rational experience.

May Week proceeded in its usual vein, parties, parties, and more parties. The feeling of being cut off from it all persisted, but I did try to seek some form of advice from a few people. Through them I resolved to write to Rachel and then get down to see her as soon as I could. This would take a few days, but there seemed to be little other option. It seemed that I couldn't just let it rest and that I should try to do something to rescue the situation, or at the very least, find out where she was coming from. The surprise of it all and the lack of any understanding of why she had taken this course of action continued to weigh heavily in my thinking. I penned a carefully written letter and sent it saying I would be down in a few days. I think deep down, I knew already that this would be a fruitless exercise, but I had to do something. At least if I knew why, maybe I would be able to move on, however difficult it would prove to be.

I was due in the area to sing the following week but I felt it would be much easier to meet before then and come down a second time the next week. I arranged for somewhere to stay whilst at one of the many parties of May Week which proved to be less than ideal, but I did make it down in the end, keeping my real purpose to myself. The deception was already in operation at that early stage. It seemed an overwhelming need to keep it all to myself as much as I possibly could. Maybe that was a mistake, but it was one that I continued to make over the years. Perhaps if I hadn't, things would have turned out a different way.

The journey down was a maelstrom of emotion. I knew that this would be the only chance of saving things, but I didn't hold out a great deal of hope. As people tend to do, I rehearsed all possibilities mentally during the journey; the good outcome, the bad, any form of compromise if one were possible. The thought processes were very strong as I drove down to the South Coast. Fear, anticipation, trepidation, they all filled my thoughts at one stage or another. Yet still that detached feeling, that mental repetition of what had transpired on the first Saturday of May Week. We met in a Wine Bar near the sea. Met up, but not alone. It seemed an omen of what was to come, but the others I knew well and they were to be trusted. In retrospect she just needed to have some sort of moral support, someone to turn the conversation to afterwards.

A Pillar of Impotence

"Thanks for your letter," was her first comment. Then the damning line, "I'm not going to change my mind." It was over before anything had been said. There was no way back this time. That was the only meaningful thing she had to say all afternoon. Then it was just back to the crass banter people tend to indulge in when out in a bar. Meaningless nothing, with which people pass their staid lives most of the time. It was over without anything else to be said. Nothing I said or did would make the slightest difference, a totally hopeless situation.

She had changed dramatically. It was as if I were talking to someone hiding behind a veil, a plastic screen, like those apparently popular in the American penal system. We could talk rationally and intelligently, but there was no reality to it. There was no way through on any form of emotional level. She'd completely closed her mind to me. I got the impression that she feared that I might talk her into doing something her head told her not to do, and she completely refused to be drawn into anything that was not on a superficial level; there was no explanation of why, perhaps for those reasons. I'd been aware from the moment we got together that I represented someone outside of the world her Faith allowed. I was completely different to the people in her rather ordered world, and maybe that was why we'd been drawn together. Who I was in public, and who I was in private had always been an issue she had wrestled with. Her response seemed to be to shut her mind down to me completely. It protected her, but damaged me more. What I felt I needed was some form of an explanation. It was never forthcoming although we would be in touch for many years after. It was always quite obvious that she cared, but she wouldn't let me into anything about her feelings for another year. She just closed down from me emotionally. Later, there was just the occasional throw away comment in person, and a few hints of how things were going in subsequent letters. But that was in the future. The present simply made things worse. Shut out completely, with no understanding of what had happened, my mental state began to deteriorate rapidly.

For the two nights I stayed in the area, I didn't sleep at all. Passing motorists may have seen the strange sight of me in a dressing gown and boots pacing the front garden, and chain smoking as they moved through residential Hove at all hours of the night. I became completely oblivious to all around me as she haunted my mind through the night. Solitude was needed but I was always with her, never alone. She would not leave my head. I returned to Cambridge in the same vein, driving the M25 on autopilot, aware yet not aware. When I returned to sing the following week, she had gone away to visit Oxford, despite promising to see me. It seemed that the hiding continued as I sat outside the pub during the World Cup, lost in my own thoughts. David Platt scoring a late winner against Belgium, and the subsequent eruption of noise caused barely a stir in my musings. The partying went on long into the night for England supporters, but I was just on the periphery, simply going through the motions. She'd run for the first time, and I knew no more now than I had on that first Saturday.

The following day the results of the Part I History Tripos were published. Results were posted on boards at the Senate House in the centre of Cambridge. It was a building I'd known for many years, having on several occasions sung at Honourary Degree Ceremonies there as a child. It was the building in which Cambridge degrees were conferred in a bizarre and archaic ceremony for those who made it through their three or four years of study. One would then return some years after to receive the equally archaic Cambridge Masters degree, allowing one to use the unlikely title of M.A. (Cantab). It was a title either misunderstood, laughed at, or resented by some who hadn't been to Oxford or Cambridge. Really it was just an excuse to get together for dinner and drinking for nostalgia's sake; a chance to reminisce about the past when life had become more real later. Although results were published at the Senate House, few undergraduates were ever there to see them. In their zeal to get on with the conference season, or in some cases to prevent revelling students damaging property, College authorities had usually removed undergraduates from College well before results were actually published. So it proved that that year, and indeed the following year for Part II of the Tripos, I was not there to see the boards at the Senate House.

At the time I had a friendly rivalry with an old school friend. Steve had gone to university in the north of England whilst I had gone to Cambridge. We met up often, usually at singing events, and undertook verbal jousting contests on the relative merits of our respective institutions on such occasions. On the surface we had little in common, save that we were both good at our chosen subjects, and sang together. It always seemed that we just joked with each other, but inside, the rivalry was rather more serious than either of us would care to admit publicly. Both of us craved the achievement of getting a first, then the argument would return to which institution was better, and the relative value of the different awards. Steve was to be one of my companions for the proposed holiday to France in August, and we planned to book it that day or the day after. He had been with me at the concert, although he knew nothing of the turmoil I faced. He was with me that day, and he had also already got his first that year.

I had no access to a phone and was forced to use a pay phone, one of those old ones where the sounds of both participants in the conversation have a habit of reverberating around the box itself. I called my Director of Studies late in the morning, with a mixture of anticipation, and some trepidation. I desperately wanted the first, but knew equally that nothing in an exam is ever certain. We exchanged the usual pleasantries at the start of the conversation, and he gave nothing away at that stage. Then his voice became rather sullen and grave as we got to the business part of the conversation.

"I think you are going to be disappointed", he started. There was a brief but interminable pause. With great speed, my mind thought through the connotations of the comment, "disappointed" is, of course, an entirely subjective concept. Then came the second part of the sentence; "you got a 2:2". The words quite literally echoed around the box, continuing to do so in my thoughts over and over again. It was as if I was mentally recreating the physical echo of what had been said.

The rest of conversation was eradicated from my mind almost the moment it had been concluded. No doubt it was polite, with many consolations offered, but it was entirely irrelevant in my eyes, and remained for no more than a few seconds in my memory. I was completely stunned; the thought of getting a 2:2 had never even crossed my mind. Maybe arrogance or misplaced blind faith had let me down; or maybe I had been deluding myself. I wanted to know what had happened, but at the same time, I knew it would make no difference to how I felt. The entire trilogy had fallen in just a few days. The world had ceased to be the same the moment it was over with Rachel, but this was another terrible blow. It later transpired that I had fallen foul of the peculiar way in which Cambridge chose to classify its History Tripos exams; had it been classified on a percentage basis, as seems to happen with so many exams, I would have had a reasonable 2:1. Not enough for me, but not this bad.

Whatever the explanations, the result stood, not only on paper, but more importantly, in my own mind. The cock had crowed thrice as the biblical phrase put it, and as it crowed each time, the betrayal of me became worse. It was not a betrayal by others but by me. I had to face Steve a few minutes later. He was, like many were to be in the next few years, completely lost as to what to say to me. I was just as lost as to what to do, my thinking on a different plane to before. I also had to return home for that long holiday that I had always dreaded so. I drove home in mental turmoil, knowing the chronic isolation I was about to face until the following October. Two days later my cat was run over and killed. Just another event that was to become the norm for me from now on.

The summer proved to be utterly horrific. My already strained relationship with my family was completely destroyed. I retreated into a world only known to myself. I was no longer able or willing to keep up the pretence that had always been required to live at home. I'd always been almost chameleon like in my ability to be whatever I was required to be depending on the surroundings in which I found myself. Now I no longer had the energy or inclination to pretend to be what I was not. I couldn't be bothered to keep the peace, and play the dutiful son any more. The response I got was to be treated as some sort of self centred outcast. Although it had been noticed that things had changed, nobody seemed to care what was happening, just about the perceived selfishness I was apparently showing. The truth was probably the complete reverse. I was just desperately trying to hang on to whatever was left of me. It just seemed to slip away as each day slipped by, and I could see no one to turn to for help.

The thoughts just kept going in on themselves, and at the centre of these was always Rachel. That was what mattered above anything else. Even this early, I had ceased to have much control over them. Although it was not until over two years later that I was able pin down what was happening, she was already talking to me in that quiet echoing voice, just as the voices had echoed in that phone box.

The voice got louder and more intense the more I thought. The contact we had over the summer remained in the same veiled falsity it had been, although it seemed, at least temporarily, to lift me. There were also several opportunities of escape that I took as often as I could, but I always had to come back home. And Rachel always came with me.

Very soon after the start of the holidays, I went up to Cambridge for a few days. One of my tutors had arranged for me to stay in guest rooms at his college for a couple of days. He was as stunned as I was about the Tripos results. As he put it: "I looked at the list of firsts, looked at the 2:1s, looked back at the firsts and thought it was a misprint". We thought about appealing but decided that that may do more harm than good. Whatever happened, I was stuck with this. We dined grandly, supped copiously, and had the usual good time. We went to Grantchester, a place that had many happy memories for me. But my perception of Cambridge had moved as well. I had always regarded the place as my real home, having spent so much of my rather fraught childhood there. Unlike Grantchester, it did have some bad memories, but it was still home. I had felt that if anything could bring about a change in my mood, it would be to go back there. But it all carried on as it was at home. Nothing changed, a fact that concerned me greatly. Wherever I went, the sensation and all that it entailed followed me. I would later describe it as "itinerant madness". But that form of sense was yet to come. No one knew then that I was ill, or how ill I was, or indeed quite how much worse it was to get. I had the knowledge that something was very wrong, but I had no idea what it was or that it was to be given a number of different names as the weeks of disorientation turned into years. Whatever I did, the pain was with me.

In between trips, life took on a morose reality. In previous holidays I had had a job working in a small factory to which I had been invited back in the future. That summer the coming recession had already hit hard at such small manufacturing concerns, and I was unable to go back. There simply wasn't enough work to keep them going. It was a sign of things to come in the early 1990s, but in Cambridge we were largely cocooned from that side of life. Few of us realised how bad things were going to get for people of all backgrounds; we still all blundered on in the wake of the late 1980s and all that Thatcherism had brought to the supposed educational elite. It caused many problems at home, and of course, kept me around the house more than I wanted. I took to taking very long walks most of the day, which brought me yet more time to be with my thoughts. I used to blindly read the property pages of the newspapers in some naive hope that my money could get me away from there for a couple of months.

A few weeks into that summer, I went to a suitably grand party at a country house. I had been rather shocked to discover that it was marked on the map. Although I'd come into contact with a number of wealthy friends over the years, I'd never been to anything quite like this before. It was also the first time that I met up with the Cambridge crowd since the end of term. The party was very much as I expected; a great deal of grandeur, good food, and huge amounts to drink. But I felt completely lost there, cut off from everyone. I'd asked Rachel if she wanted to come while we were still together, but she had said she would feel out of place there. Now I felt exactly as she had anticipated she'd feel; with the people I wanted to be with most, but cut off from them. I found my self alone by the pool at one stage, surrounded by night candles. In the flickering light they offered, I was physically alone but Rachel was there in my head. For the first time in years I wept. Uncontrollable and unexplained tears. I stayed in my loneliness for over an hour. When I returned, I don't think anyone had noticed my absence. I just carried on the pretence, drank more, and knew I'd have to return home the next day.

The summer drifted along in much the same way, and I waited impatiently for the holiday to come. My interest was briefly sparked by the invasion of Kuwait in the first week of August, but that interest was merely confined to reading the papers in the morning and watching the nightly news bulletins. A couple of weeks later we set off to France, and at last I had what I hoped would be a two week period of sustained absence, not only from home, but also my troubled mind. It was of course a vain and delusionary hope. We crossed the Channel to Dieppe and spent two weeks driving south taking in many of the historic towns and cities, culminating in the rather obscure city of Mende with its vast Cathedral and very little else, before returning via Cluny and Fecamp.

With the exception of the remnants of the monastery at Cluny, very few of the places even registered any interest for me. They were just places of which I knew, but from which I was completely detached. Whilst Steve and Neil took great pleasure from the sites and buildings I mainly adjourned to the nearest bar to drink coffee in the day, and beer at night. Both beverages were inevitably accompanied by endless cigarettes and damaging contemplation. I usually shared a twin room with Steve on the journey, and unknown to him, would sit up until the dawn thinking and smoking through the open window. As expected nothing changed in my mind, it was just that the surroundings were rather more beautiful than, and different from the tedium of the South coast. It was on one of these late night sojourns that the tears returned. It was just as unexpected and unexplained as at the country house; and just as disturbing. I knew that life was falling apart if it hadn't done so already, but it just seemed such a strange reaction to have. For the first time that night I thought that I was having a breakdown, but then I couldn't work out what the phrase meant. It's one used so commonly by people but few consciously consider exactly what it is. I dismissed it out of hand as I was wont to do with things that I did not understand. Steve slept on in oblivion.

There were moments of joy but these were short lived and closely linked to the amount we drank, a pattern that was to recur frequently over the years. The mood turned further into the depths as we headed back for the journey north. The end of the escape, however superficial it had proved to be, loomed large on that journey. I had come to the definite decision that I was going to give up singing on my return to Cambridge. And I knew the implications that would have for the already destroyed relations with my family. I had that joy to face back in England as well as all the other mechanics that now comprised my mental state. None of it had changed in the time I was away, but then it had always been a hope that I knew I could never attain by two weeks abroad. Rachel was still dominating my mind, and there was still another month and a week to go before I could seek my refuge back in Cambridge; and Cambridge meant finals along with it all.

On my return I was immediately engulfed in wedding preparations. My sister was to be married on the 1st of September. Before then though was the small matter of my 21st birthday, and I'd not been overly enamoured of the idea of her marrying two days later, knowing that it would prove be a side show to the main event. I'd always hated having a birthday at the end of the holidays because I never had the chance to see any friends. It was also usually in the August Bank holiday week so every few years it fell on that weekend, and there was no post. As a very young child I had forlornly sat on the verge outside the house waiting for the post that was destined never to arrive. When I was older and singing, I was often abroad which was better, but also brought other problems such as lengthy rehearsals and concerts on the day, and potentially, violence. Now I faced the prospect of facing that mythically symbolic day alone with my family, and overshadowed by the forthcoming event. I did receive many cards that day but felt it was all very contrived, people only doing it because they were aware of what was to come. Despite the protestations to the contrary by others, the day was, as expected, awful, and quickly forgotten by all but me; another little event that was to play havoc with my mind.

The wedding passed off relatively uneventfully. The only interruption being when my mother nearly caused a scene by declaring that I was supposed to be driving them home after when I had specifically made it clear that we were going to get a cab the day before. It was merely what I had come to expect. We did return by cab and she told me that I should recoup the cost from my sister. I didn't.

Within a few days, I was off on my travels again, this time down to Sussex to spend time with a variety of school friends for a couple of weeks. The relay that had been suggested whilst at school was put into operation, only on a smaller scale than had originally been envisaged. This did not go down well at home, but I had long since ceased to give a shit about that, it was just another temporary escape. I saw Rachel during this time; she was pleasant enough but still veiled from me. She seemed oblivious to the damage that had been caused; she either genuinely didn't know or she hid herself from it, refusing to acknowledge it. I couldn't tell which, but I noticed that her Faith and religious view had become much more overt and public. There had been a change in her, just as there had in me; religion had been a much more private thing than it was now. I wondered if that was significant.

A Pillar of Impotence

The summer finally ended. I still had no solutions; I was still utterly confused; nothing made a great deal of sense. More importantly, I had become even more isolated, and was almost completely estranged from my parents. I had resolved that if things worked out and I made it through the next year and got away, I would endeavour never to see them again. We'd never been a family in my eyes, and what there was, was now completely destroyed.

As I returned home to my refuge, I reflected on the hell that had been that summer.

Chapter 4

Final Refuge

For too many people, the realisation of the finality of that last year at university came alarmingly late in the day. Three years is but a brief moment in the lives that many are destined to lead; at 18 years old when one is about to embark on a university course, that idea is hard to conceptualise. For those able enough, and lucky enough to go down that route, life through education is pretty much mapped out up until that final year. Primary school, secondary school, jumping through the right hoops at the prescribed time, and then on to university. But in that final year, the map peters out, there are to be no more grants or loans, and real choices have to be made. After the fun we had in the first two years, this realisation came as something of a jolt for many. Many more failed to realise how hard it was about to prove in that particular year.

In the late 1980s when we had come to Cambridge, graduates were in high demand. The "Milk Round" operated where the employers came to you when the last year as an undergraduate started. People left to find employment in many fields at often ridiculous starting salaries. The last years of Thatcherism had been good for those who wanted to, and indeed lived to make money. For the first two years we'd lived with this legacy, the expectation being that it would be relatively easy to move on, and above all, be able to make a great deal of money. That was the ideal on which many of us had been brought up; better and more education would lead to better jobs and more money. The revival from the recession and unemployment of the early 1980s had been based on such principals. Having grown up with that, it had a great deal to do with why people tried to go to Oxford and Cambridge. The "Milk Round" was one means by which this was facilitated. That year, it never took place; virtually every company pulled out as recession returned to the country with all the consequences that it could bring.

As I returned for the third year, this was all in the future, and to me, utterly irrelevant. I knew, even then, that it was a going to be a fight just to get through. The emotional mauling that I had suffered that summer was still very much with me, even though I had returned, at last, to the one place that I desperately wanted to be.

I moved into a house belonging to the college with a couple of friends. It was a large house on the edge of the college grounds. We shared it with five other students, and the room of the Director of Music, the man to whom I had to announce my retirement from singing at some stage soon. There was a large kitchen table around which there were to be many giant breakfasts for others, and the inevitable house parties. The bathrooms upstairs overlooked the playing field on which I had played so much school rugby and football as a child; opposite the school where I had first ventured into the realms of serious singing. Now I was to give that up; it had served its purpose as an aid to getting back to Cambridge for real.

Despite the large kitchen, we were still close to college, and the inherent ease that the Dining Hall afforded us. Later, we did turn our collective hands to the idea of self catering on the grounds that it would save our dwindling resources; on those grounds the idea failed dismally as we hung on the curious opulence of Cambridge, competing with one another on the culinary front. As a means of enjoyment, it was a great success. The house was also ideally suited to the pursuit of Part II of the History Tripos; the building next door was the Faculty of Music; the one next to that, set a little back from the road, was the infamous Sealey Library, seat of the study of history at the University of Cambridge. So to actually get there merely required falling out of the front door and crossing a car park. This requirement was much in evidence as we entered the third year; history students, famed for the lack of set times to work, were actually required to do something in Part II of the course. Having been to six lectures in two years, I now had to attend with some regularity, although those of a more scientific bent still laughed at the timetable we were set. Not only did we have to attend, but it also required getting up before 11 o' clock, so at the house we were ideally placed to roll in the door just about on time.

I came to love that house as time began to run out on Cambridge. It was to become a symbol of refuge as time began to slowly disappear, and I knew that what awaited me at the end would make the summer that had just passed pale into insignificance. From the start I knew that it was to be just a temporary respite, and of course all that had gone on in my mind was destined to continue, in-spite of the change of venue. Rachel still dominated. For the first time I began to find the work harder. It wasn't that the course was any harder, it was just that it was now so hard to focus, to get motivated. What had seemed so easy in the first two years now seemed to drag me down, a distraction to what was really going on. Again, I seemed to be just going through the motions, although I did retain a sense that it needed to get done; I had to maintain myself in my spiritual home for as long as I could.

I duly gave up singing, with the slight misgivings that I had let them down by not making contact earlier. I was asked to put it into writing, but, even though all that was required was to scribble a note and take it downstairs, I could never bring myself to do it; just as I couldn't be bothered to get in touch before; it seemed such an effort for something that mattered so little. As expected the reaction of my parents was bad; they were left no longer able to social climb on the back of my singing abilities. That is how it had always been; nothing else mattered to them apart from music. But I had to give it up to take over the American Football team; at least that was something I had a great passion for. Music had always been a means to an end, not something I greatly enjoyed. It had got me to where I wanted to be, although I'd paid a price unknown to anyone. Living where I did, there were constant reminders of that immediately over the road.

From the start, however, things began to go seriously wrong in the Football world. Having made the decision to join the Universities League the previous summer, I returned to find that hardly anyone wanted to play; I had about half a dozen players, and only three weeks until the first game. It just went from bad to worse as promises of kit failed to materialise, leading to me having to pay for it. I was plunged into a constant battle to find new players, and to chase those who might come back. Why don't people bother to contact me either way? That became another constant in my over crowded thinking, along with all that had happened previously.

In spite of the problems which were to continue all season, playing the game was the only thing that made me happy. Sport had always been my release from the pressures of singing; now it became the only thing that kept me going. Through all the troubles and stress it caused me, it was also my lifeline. I kept having rather dark thoughts as to what would happen if the team folded. On many occasions I got to the point where I felt I couldn't carry on; I was a terrible delegator, but didn't trust anyone else to do it for me. Deep down I knew how serious it would be for me to lose it, although my mind stopped me short of what the ultimate consequences would be; suicide was the hidden unspeakable concept at that stage, and my mind wouldn't yet let me near that thought.

Having fought so hard to get things going, I suffered a personal catastrophe when I tore a muscle in my leg quite early in the first match, and was most unlikely to be able to play again before Christmas. It also stopped me playing rugby. I was left with all the hard and dull part of organisation, and none of the enjoyment. My release from pain was gone.

Not withstanding these problems, and not the least of these was the difficulty of getting about, life went on as normal. At least that was the public face of it. Privately I was disintegrating. I was often struck by how fake life had become. Many times a day we are asked the rather closed question of "How are you?" Few answer with the truth or in more than a one word response. As I was asked this question, I kept thinking to myself that I was very far from alright, the answer I invariably gave. This was the first genuine realisation that something was going seriously wrong. This idea became another mainstay of my thinking. I also continued to muse on the idea of what exactly a breakdown was. Often I felt I must be having one, but continued to dismiss the idea as an anomaly; if I didn't understand what it was, it was dismissed.

Along with these thoughts came the idea that perhaps I should go and see a Doctor. Maybe they will be able to tell me what is going on. More active thinking. Again I dismissed the idea on the assumption that they would tell me that it was just stress at the thought of the forthcoming Finals. Knowing as I did that that was far removed from the root of the problem, I never went. Subsequent events were to prove that conviction to have been correct. I was always aware from the moment it started what the root cause was, and I also knew that the real point would be missed. There was always insight, just no solution that would ease the situation.

On some occasions I spoke to those around me, most notably to a friend whose boyfriend had died in unexpected circumstances in the first year. There was much sympathy, but little concrete help beyond the standard idea of letting go and moving on.

People cared but that was not enough. The isolation and detachment I had felt over the summer continued and got worse, even around those I wished to be with. I continued on the college social scene with aplomb, but was increasingly uncomfortable with it. I would often just be there, engrossed in my thoughts, saying what was required, but not really there. Often my thoughts turned to my former colleague, the one we'd all lost about 18 months before. There was a great sense of fakeness in all that was around. With that came the idea that I was a fake. What am I doing here? How did I get here? I don't deserve to be here. I've conned my way in here. Who am I? The thoughts became increasingly uncontrollable.

The constant thought took its toll on my real one escape, sleep. Insomnia began to set in. My mood became increasingly erratic, although I rarely, if ever, displayed that in public. Although I was constantly preoccupied and down, on occasion, the mood would slump even lower for no apparent reason. I could understand reacting to things going wrong, particularly with the Football club, but the sudden shifts made no sense. It was as if there was a switch somewhere in my head that was flicked without any control or reason. Once it happened, there was nothing I could do to alleviate the feelings.

My response to the increasing despair that I felt was to go out and spend money. Although I had more than many, it was finite in quantity, and the Football club was proving an expensive proposition that I was effectively underwriting. But I had to do it just to keep going. Much was spent eating well and drinking. Each occasion though provided but a brief respite for me. At the same time my need for coffee and cigarettes went up dramatically, as did that for alcohol. The relief that such drugs brought was always temporary. As often as I drank, I always knew that when I awoke, it would all be the same again. But at least the alcohol helped me to sleep and drove away the constant thought processes. That was one of the few blessings that I had.

A Pillar of Impotence

I sat in my room one Sunday night late in that term watching the NFL on my tiny, and elderly black and white TV. The tears returned. Unexpected as they had been on the previous occasions, this time it was worse. How could it happen when I was indulging myself in one of the few distractions I had? It made no sense but continued. I heard a knock at the door, and the voice of a friend. I hid myself away, the pretence that I was not there. I just couldn't face it. No one could know how much pain I was in. It confirmed to me that things had reached an alarmingly bad point. It also confirmed my need to keep it well hidden. It was what I'd known all my life. I'd always hidden my self from the world around, at least what really mattered, and who I really was. Perhaps foolishly, I determined to keep to what I knew. It never seriously crossed my mind to seek help mainly because I knew there was little hope of getting it; at least what I really needed and I didn't know what that was.

Somehow, I made it through the term. At the Christmas Ball I met someone from the past, someone I'd not seen for years. I had no idea what to say to him, or any interest in talking to him. I was just too detached. I drank copiously, but was mentally shut down from all around me. Then I had to return home to even greater isolation.

I have no memory of that Christmas and New Year. It has just been wiped from my mind. Supposition inevitably suggests that it was even worse than the summer had been. There were only two terms to go after that. The sands were slowly slipping away for me, as time moved on.

The new term brought a general sense of unease and despair throughout the members of my year. The disappearance of the "Milk Round" had brought with it a great deal of uncertainty. Many who had had no previous interest in the Law or Accountancy found themselves headed down that road. There was little else to do. Others desperately scrambled for places on Postgraduate courses to try to ride out the storm of recession that had seized the country. My despair was rather more personal. I had no idea what I wanted to do, but that was the least of my concerns. I was reduced to just trying to get through each day and ultimately to get the degree. Heady thoughts of trying to get back the first I had missed the year before had long since disappeared from my mind.

Mid January also brought the start of the Gulf War. The feeling of patriotism for a while distracted many from their own problems. It had quite a profound effect on the mood of the public, and for a while served its purpose. I was distracted, but only in a very limited way. Rachel became increasingly loud, her voice a many times a day occurrence. We still had real contact, and I had seen her on few occasions. Still the same guarded and veiled demeanour. The only place she was real was in my thoughts and in my head, and that wasn't real. Real or not, I could do nothing to stop her.

The Football club remained a constant fight for me, but one I had to keep going with. Bad weather delayed my return to the field, and when I did, more physical ailments plagued me. But it was a relief to get back to doing the one thing genuinely distracted me. I also had to prepare for the forthcoming Varsity Bowl. More problems to iron out. More stress. It just kept getting more difficult to keep up with. But I had to keep going.

I returned to the river for the Lent Bumps. We put together what is quaintly known as a "Gentlemen's Eight", the traditional turn up on the day crew that races in the lower divisions for fun. It was often a way to get Blades as experienced rowers could come up against weaker opposition, albeit from the point of view of being very unfit and out of practise. The danger was that other such boats could linger in the lower reaches of the pecking order, trying to do exactly the same thing. It was an unpredictable adventure for all involved. Fun though it was, we were caught in that position and did not get Blades. For me it was an attempt at retrieving an irretrievable situation. It failed. Had we achieved our Blades, it is very doubtful that it would have been much of a consolation for me. Just another thing to do in a life that was already far beyond my capacity to deal with.

A week later, we were beaten in the Varsity Bowl. Amazingly enough, my family had actually decided to come and watch. They seemed to enjoy it, but my mother was somewhat shocked by the violence and danger of the game. We had a good night after with the team, but the next day I took to my bed for the first time in years. It seemed like having a three day hangover. In reality, it was complete physical and mental exhaustion. The problems that running the team had thrown in my direction were gone. I had survived a situation that had very nearly broken me. It had seemed that everything that could go wrong did. The final failure was that we were never able to get the whole team together for a club dinner; nor did we ever manage a complete team photo. It kept going wrong, even to the end. Although the stress was now gone, so was my one reason to keep going. I was left in an empty void, a vacuum where my only companion was my thoughts. With those thoughts came Rachel, ever stronger, and harder now to counteract.

Right at the end of term, I made a belated attempt to try to sort something out for the following year. I applied to do a Masters Degree in International Relations. It was a course many of my Football colleagues from the States were doing. Much paper work had to be got through applying for the course and the funding, and I had to put together a research proposal. As I was not able to stay in the house outside of term, I stayed with my sister a few miles away for a while, and commuted in. The house was alarmingly empty as I sat working on the kitchen table. The door was locked, something that never happened when we were there. I was struck by the loneliness of it all as I worked. It just seemed one task too many for me. My mind was so distracted that I struggled to focus; I was too tired even to think straight. With some liaison with various tutors, I finally managed to get it all sorted. It was to prove to have been a great effort in vain. I'd applied too late, the course being full although the closing date had not expired. Maybe next year. I knew I would never make it to that point, and I needed something now. In the end, I would never have even got the funding; that was dependant on getting that elusive first. That was never going to happen now. Since Part I, I had struggled with the idea of what exactly did I have to do to get a good grade; now it was a case of whether I'd make it through at all.

Since that day in June I'd been through a great deal; attended two more Boat Club dinners; run the American Football; played in my third Varsity Bowl, something no one else in Cambridge had done; given up singing; returned to the river, failing once again to get the Blades; got through the work as best I could; and above all else had wrecked myself both physically and mentally. Still I could find no way forward or out of it. The future held finals, another Boat Club Dinner, another Ball and Suicide Sunday; and Graduation would follow that, if I made it. Then there was just a great abyss. My time in my refuge was nearly over.

Chapter 5

Asylum Runs Out

The Easter holidays were mercifully short, although in the grand scheme of time slipping away, this time it was little consolation. There was, however, going to be one final distraction; Easter in Spain. Although I'd given up singing regularly in Cambridge, I still occasionally sang and toured elsewhere. A trip abroad at or around Easter had long been a habit of mine; one I relished and cultivated as another means of escape. Although in many respects singing had long since become a tedious job, it had taken me too many places over the years. Unlike the monotony of holding the Choral Exhibition in Cambridge, these external trips were as much social occasions as anything else. The singing was taken seriously but above all, we enjoyed the places we went to. I had toured in Cambridge, but that had been the same job like atmosphere, with a load of people who were overwhelmingly only interested in music. That was the least of my interests, and that trip had been something of a let down for me. Now Spain loomed large as final anchor point before the coming, and by then, anticipated catastrophe that was about to engulf me.

My studies of the Crown of Aragon fitted in quite well with going to Barcelona, it having been the capital of their empire. The singing at various places in the area would allow me to see some of the sites with which I was to have to become so familiar in the next couple of months. How much historical value it would be was something of a moot point, but I did hope to have a chance to see the Crown Records housed in the Cathedral. On the basis of this rather tenuous theory, I had applied to the college for a travel grant. The application was successful, and a modest amount sent to me by cheque. Although the cost of the trip was relatively small it was very helpful; resources were dwindling rapidly after the exertions of funding the Football Club, and the desperate attempts I had made since the summer to spend my way to some sort of stability. That aside, I was determined to make the most of what was looking likely to be the last trip before the ensuing chaos of post graduation life.

Having struggled through the first week or so of the holidays, I set off for the trip trying to set aside the grave problems that beset me. Although many people on the trip knew Rachel, she was not there; at least not in body but only in my mind. Few knew of the turmoil or my feelings, and for the most part I got through without her being an open issue. The tour lived up to its usual expectations with a great deal of partying. It was a time to meet up with many old friends, and to make new acquaintances. I simply switched into a kind of May Week mode, and, as best I could, enjoyed the occasion. There remained the sense of falseness throughout, and as the week progressed, I found myself counting off the days, knowing as I did what was to come. It was only at the end, when we had returned to this country that I made things apparent to one of the new people I'd met. We had a wonderful dinner in which for the first time I was able to open up and talk, dispelling the myth that I had purveyed all week. The meeting was cut short, but for a short fleeting time, I felt at ease with myself; the first time I felt that maybe there was support out there. Sophie was to remain one of my great supporters over the years, but a supporter who was at a loss as to what to do. Frustrating though it was for both of us that impotence was to mark the support that I received from many as time went by, and things got progressively worse. It was a first step, one that would be repeated many times as more and more people made it through to the peculiarities that were to become the norm for me. I often felt that I shouldn't let people into such a world. At the same time, I desperately need them, however little they offered in terms of concrete help. Guilt would often descend after, the feeling that I couldn't burden others with my needs.

I went home for one night before going back to Cambridge. Spain had been a much better distraction than France had been the previous year. Although Rachel had been with me all the time, and there were constant reminders of her in the people around me, I managed to put her to the background for much of the time. Like all distractions though, they are by definition, temporary. As I sat at home, I mused on what was to come. I watched *A Room With A View* that night. As I watched, a tremendous sense of calm overtook me. A calm I'd not known for months. I was physically exhausted from the trip, and emotionally drained by the last few months, but that passed away with the calm. I knew that the next day I had to travel for the final time to my place of refuge. I knew also that I had to steel myself for what awaited me on my return. In this unusual calm these thoughts went back and forth, but were lost and conquered. For just a short time I found myself at peace. I'd forgotten what that was like. Even Rachel was quiet. That quiet continued as I slipped easily into sleep. A calm before the coming torrents of pain that I knew awaited me with the next day, and those that followed.

The journey seemed arduous, and I found an empty house when I arrived, but at least I was home. People arrived over the next day or two, and having sorted our selves out, we got down to the business that was to take so much of our time. It all boiled down to a few weeks, all those years of education culminated in this, then on to the fight as to what to do next. But that latter experience would be entirely dependent on the former, futures shaped by a few days of sitting in exam halls for three hours at a time. My concentration had weakened so much I doubted I'd even be able to last that length of time. At the same time I knew that it had to be done, so I threw myself into it as best as I could.

The most pressing problem was to catch up on all the reading that I'd singularly failed to do up to that point in the year. Life settled down into an endless round of reading and noting of set texts; the *Chronicle of James I of Aragon*; Ramon Llull's *Ars*, and the *Three Wise Men*. The list went on, each had to be laboriously read and noted, and, due to a lack of copies of some of the texts, we had a time limited rota system which limited availability. Each day started with a large pot of coffee, packets of cigarettes, the arm chair, and a text. All day this persisted, along with other revision. Coffee and cigarettes became my closest friends. The consumption grew by the day, 40, 50, and 60. With each rise came extra cost. I wound up drinking 25 cups of coffee in a day, wired to the hilt as I fought against the confines of time. I've got to get it done. Must do more tomorrow. Only two days left with James I. Thoughts crowding. Rachel was there in the background, thoughts and noises that I had to fight back.

The excesses of stimulants took their toll. Sleep became even scarcer. Alcohol, pain killers, weed, all needed to counteract the effects of the day's exertions. It never seemed to stop, but I had to keep going. I knew it was destroying me but I had no choice. I took to taking long walks alone along the river. It alleviated some of the pressure, but with it brought thoughts of Rachel and what was to happen afterwards, if I made it that far. Time was running out and still there were no solutions. Desperation grew by the day, an endless cycle of things to do, few of which offered much relief.

There were to be some occasions of joy, ones that brought back the old days, if only for a short while. Sophie came to visit for a couple of days and we resumed the interrupted conversation of post Easter; a release of sorts. Others came too, and I slowly began to bring things out into the open. The process continued with a few Cambridge people. Those around me were alarmed about the future, the recession causing so many problems. We often joked about living in Cardboard City, so bad was the situation. I had that to contend with as well but it was what was going in my head that was most alarming. Although I'd dedicated myself, at great physical and emotional cost to getting through, I knew that what awaited me at the end was too frightening to think about. For all the escapes the thought of breakdown was upper most in my mind. Through all this I often wondered what a shrink would make of me. Quiet and private musings, but sub consciously, I knew that was probably what was in stall for me after.

On the 11th May, we held what was to prove to be the best party in the three years of Cambridge. Sitting in the bar the previous night, it was decided that we should have a party the following day; through all the pressure, decadence was to be our watch word right to the end. So was born the Bob Marley Memorial Party. Invites to a barbecue were printed that night for an evening of Red Stripe, food, and wall to wall Marley. With stereo and fridge in the garden, we entertained in our usual fashion. As expected, we were closed down by the porters for not asking permission, but the effect was magical. Probably the greatest night we had in all our time there. As one of our guests said afterwards "it was the only party that you didn't feel you needed to get pissed at". A marvellous diversion and one I tried very hard to hang on to. It worked in limited way. The next day I still had to wake up to the chaos that now inhabited my mind.

Over the course of the term, conciliatory noises started to come from Rachel. I saw her on occasion, and although the veil was always there, the signs seemed good. I knew it would never get back to where it was before, but maybe I might get an explanation that would help. Whether it was the reports she'd had from those who had seen me or something else, she decided that she wanted to come to Cambridge for a few days after exams. It was a prospect I looked forward to, and dreaded in equal measure. I could see no harm in it, and potentially some good. I still clung to the idea that if I could understand what had happened, maybe the fears of the future could be avoided or lessened.

In my rare bits of spare time, I finally started to write about what seemed to be going on. I pondered on my own sanity. Things had long since ceased to make any sense in my life, so maybe that was it. I rambled away in my own way, some of it making sense, other bits not. Maybe I was trying to bring some sense to things, but if that was the case, it failed. It just went on and on endeavouring to explain the unexplainable. It was the first time I'd ever written about myself and my feelings, but brought me little comfort, just a testimony to what I perceived was happening. It was as if I'd lost all belief or concept as to what self was, a writing down of some of this myriad of perpetual thoughts that I couldn't stop. I often wondered why I was bothering but I managed to keep going without much purpose. I suppose though that it was an escape from work, just as my river walks to Grassy were a physical escape.

The weeks ticked away to early June, and with them came the start of those Finals. The future was to be decided in a few short days. The days were short but the hours were long. Each exam took a mental and physical toll. Sitting for three hours was always uncomfortable, the discomfort compounded by cramping up of writing hands. I struggled to focus and remember what I needed to know and get down on paper. Each exam went past with only a hint of relief. Although it was good to get each out of the way, the relief was tinged with the thought that that was one step closer to the end. Our year was the first to experience the tribulations of having to do a general paper as part of Finals. We had had to do one in Part I, and great consternation was felt when it was announced that we had to do it again. So much fuss was caused that it was agreed that it wouldn't count towards our marks, but we still had to do it. Three hours, one essay on a general concept that I failed entirely to understand. That one, as expected, proved to be the worse of them all.

I finished my last exam at 4.30. Immediately I hurried from the Sidgewick Site, down the Avenue, and across Silver Street Bridge to the Anchor. The journey took all of five minutes from door to door. Others awaited us there with champagne. Much to my surprise, there was a face from the past as well. Behind the bar was a girl from my school days in Cambridge. Despite having been in that pub many times I had never seen her working there before. Her brother had been a friend of mine long before. He'd been dead for some years, but I still thought of him from time to time. She didn't recognise me and I let it pass, but it stuck in my mind. Another thought to contend with. The evening was monumental even by Cambridge standards. A pub crawl ensued, interrupted by Greek food and wine, the latter bringing on an early hangover before even venturing to bed. Some how we made it home eventually, the evening having long since descended into a haze rapidly erased from my memory. The next day would mark the beginning of the future. Now I had nothing to hang on to. The Football Club was over, now exams were over. What was left?

We had about two weeks to go until Graduation. Much was to come: another Ball; the Bumps; Suicide Sunday; May Week; and then the end. All that was to bring so many memories of the year before, memories of Rachel, and still no answers, just confusion.

The days of those two weeks were, in many respects, idyllic. The weather was hot, and we passed the time punting, drinking, and watching the bumps, the usual Cambridge fare. A whole group of us travelled to Alton Towers for the day, enjoying the new found, if brief freedom afforded us by the end of exams. We had some Americans to stay in the house at the time, people met by one on my colleagues whilst travelling the previous summer. It seemed to bring a strange sense of déjà vu from that summer for me, a Ball, the Bumps, and another American. It was if history was repeating in the run up to May Week. After all the pressure of the term, the rest did us all good, but as each day passed, my sense of foreboding grew. It was also getting very close to the time that I would have to go and collect Rachel as we had now finalised arrangements for her visit. Emotion started to build in me to extreme levels. Far from getting easier as the pressure was released, the constant thinking grew ever stronger. Things seemed to be coming to a head. I'd always attached great symbolism to places, dates, and times; now things seemed to be proceeding just as they had before.

The Bumps started on the Wednesday as they always did. We went to the Plough to watch on that first day. Plough Reach was always a favoured from which to watch. For a series of races where the object was to physically hit the boat in front, and to avoid being hit from behind, it was a prime spot. Coming out of the long Grassy bend and into the Reach, it was usually the site of most collisions, particularly in the lower divisions. I had decided not to Cox that term, but I knew many who did so we stayed until the last division set off in the early evening; there were fewer bumps at that level but it provided great racing. Afternoons of fine weather, a beautiful pub garden, and a great deal of Pimm's, just as it had been before. It was also opposite the place I used to take my long walks by the river. During the week, the American girl had started to take a great deal of interest in me. It was an idea that added to my overall confusion, coming as it did as we approached the anniversary of life losing its way; and of course Rachel would be there soon. The following day, in more glorious weather we repeated the process. The day after that was to be the Ball, an idea full of fear for me. More symbolism.

My sister and brother in law were coming to the Ball along with the Americans and various friends who were also to stay in the house. It promised to be a crowded and drunken night at which I would be fighting off the memories with the help of the alcohol that always flowed so freely on these occasions. During the day, we had arranged to get the Football Club photo taken. We couldn't get hold of everyone, and an unexpected Royal visit forced a rapid change of venue. Problems to the last. The photo was never even printed as we failed to get enough orders for it. It finished as it had started, on an ignominious note.

As the Ball started, the weather broke and the heavens opened; it rained all night. I spent most of that night not only dodging the rain but also the attentions of the American. I just could not cope with it on that day with all its reminiscences. Turmoil reigned in my mind. Memories of the year before came flooding back in a torrent. I fought desperately to hold them back, and above all, to keep them to myself. Balls in the rain are never a pretty sight, but fighting a past that was rapidly overtaking the present was an ugly prospect. We survived although the photo that I had missed the year before was cancelled. Soaked as we all were, after taking an early breakfast in town, everyone returned to the house to try to get some sleep before the last day of the Bumps. There was not enough room for all to sleep but I had other ideas; I needed solitude. As all slept, I slipped out of the house for another solitary walk. As the rain came again, I lay on the sodden ground and wept. With the tears Rachel's voice wreaked havoc in my head in inglorious flashback. No one knew I'd gone, and I wanted that to be so. Although I'd avoided the attentions of the girl from Ohio, it had all been so reminiscent of the previous year. It would carry on that day as yet again my parents were coming to the last day of the Bumps; and they really were the last people I wanted to see that day.

The Towpath in the rain was not a good place to be on a Saturday afternoon. As a family day it was awful. The sandy coloured mud gets everywhere, staining clothes and shoes alike, compounded by the number of bicycles passing by in pursuit of their boats. As each boat went by, the flotilla of bikes hurled drops of that mud into the air and onto those on foot. Hungover, cold, wet, and above all exhausted, I paced up and down Grassy that afternoon. My mind was anywhere but on the rowing. I was in my place of solace with people everywhere crowding my space. Symbolism of the day and what had happened the previous year overtook me mentally, just as the bikes overtook me physically. Rachel was going crazy in my head; over and over, waves of that echoing voice crashed around me. It just wouldn't stop. This was compounded by the company I was forced to endure. Where I needed to be was with the others, across the water at the Plough, and not in my overcrowded space. No one really knew how bad things were that day, but it had to be better to be with them than in my present predicament. Returning to the house after the last division had raced, the torment was partially lifted. Getting out of the wet clothes was a relief, and ushered in the move to Black Tie for yet another Boat Club Dinner. Although I had not rowed that year, there was a tradition of the Boat Club Supporters Club, a tradition I was determined to continue. It was another occasion to try to blot things out and ease things for a while. But it was still a repeat of the year before. In the oblivion that followed, I was moderately successful in achieving the aim. Yet the next day would come, and I would be back to where I had started.

A Pillar of Impotence

On Suicide Sunday the weather cleared. There was the usual scramble to find somewhere that not only would sell Pimm's before 12 o' clock, but also had sufficient stocks for our needs. We did succeed, somewhere in a back street of Newnham village. It proved to be the usual fair in the gardens of the college, bathed as they finally were in sunlight. That was a welcome change from the Ball and the Bumps. But it was also unusual that day as I finally succumbed to the American girl. History repeating. I'd spoken to her about Rachel, and the bearing that it had on me, the difficulties it placed on me where other women were concerned. It seemed mad that after a year I still couldn't go anywhere near anyone else, but that was how it was mentally. Dee had commented that "she must be mad"; I thought her comment was mad, my self belief having been so utterly taken to pieces by the events. It didn't make sense for anyone to say that. On that day I felt I had nothing to lose so I went ahead. The results were devastating to my mental state. Guilt took another turn in my overcrowded mind. That in itself made no sense but couldn't be helped. I no longer controlled what I thought or felt, and I was painfully aware that Rachel was coming to Cambridge. It was not so much regret as a sense of having made yet another huge mistake. Why did you do that? You don't deserve to have that? You've betrayed her. You were using her. Thoughts kept coming. Rachel was still at the centre of things. Now guilt was building into the deteriorating situation. I also knew that for the rest of the time Dee was in the country, I would have to keep excusing myself without appearing to be a complete shit. Life had just got immeasurably worse on that day.

The next few days took on their usual form, parties, Pimm's, and punting. May Week tended to begin at a frenetic pace, and then slow down as the days went by. It was a time to relax and enjoy the last few remnants of Cambridge life whilst trying to ignore the impending problems that were about to become all of our realities. For the most part, people were able to set aside this sense of fear; the shadow of mass unemployment was for a while overshadowed by the alternatives, however temporary they were. For me the storm was gathering a pace; for me the problems were much closer to home than what may or may not happen at some stage in the future. The world was caving in around me and there seemed no way out. Rachel was arriving within a few days, and the day after she left, Cambridge would become fleeting mirage disappearing into the distance behind me. I was soon headed to the place where there was no chance of long term escape. Had I had employment there might have been a hope, but I knew even then that I was not capable of working even if there was a job there. The money had almost run out by then; all I could see in the future was home and no money or hope to get out.

In the middle of May Week we had the Graduation Dinner. Formal and, inevitably drunken, it was an opportunity to laud our alleged success over one another. At that point I didn't know my results, but despite the problems, I felt that I had at least got through. Thoughts of getting a First were long gone, just getting through had been the focus. The thoughts of going to a Graduation Dinner and then not making it didn't really enter anyone's head as it was hard to actually fail; those who might had usually been weeded out long before that. There was the normal fair of food, wine, and passing the port in the correct direction. There were, of course, self congratulatory speeches. Students and Fellows alike spoke, and we were told what a marvellous year we had been and what a pleasure it had been for the college to have had us there for three years; more self indulgence to be lapped up by all of us. A thoroughly good evening was spoiled a couple of days later when we were told that nobody could stay in college up to the Ceremony itself, and we'd all have to go home until the day before. So much for what had been said at the Dinner. We had all expected it though. The college exists as an entity in itself; students were just a peripheral part to some within the hierarchy. There is, after all, a rapid three year turnover at such establishments; good for weeding out those who might cause trouble. Just like those in danger of failing. In addition, nothing was to happen after the Ceremony; we just had to go home then, surplus to requirements.

This decision presented me with the problem of where exactly I could stay when Rachel finally made it up. I was able to stay with a friend at another college for the couple of days of her visit, but it was far from ideal. The meeting that I anticipated and feared in equal measure would take place on unfamiliar ground. I'd known my host for many years but he had no idea what was going on in my head, or what may unfold in his house. More distractions. I arranged to go to Sussex for a few days before picking her up and bringing her back. I was then allowed to stay in the house on the night before Graduation, but no longer than that.

As I set off in the car, all I had left as it was, I left the house for almost the last time. I was venturing into the complete unknown in every way imaginable. Life had collapsed completely, and I knew that the next few days would be extremely intense. I had no idea at all how I was going to react to her presence as I left my final refuge for the penultimate time.

Chapter 6

The Veiled Lantern

The journey to Sussex took me via the gridlock of the M25 and Redhill station. I was accompanied to Redhill by one of my tutors, the one who thought I would get a First the previous year, and had been so shocked by the result. We talked of many things, both academic and social, although I gave no inkling of what the real purpose of my journey was. The gridlock was interrupted by the rather unusual experience of getting out on the motorway to give and light a cigarette to a fellow parker. As I dropped him at the station I promised to call as soon as I had my results, particularly if I had achieved anything unexpected; he still had faint hopes of the First even if I didn't. I was just hoping I'd done enough to get through. Yet again I was headed to Sussex in the days preceding the posting of results at the Senate House. The anticipation was building, the same place, the same people, the same phone box, and Rachel. The cycle that seemed to have haunted me for a year was continuing in the same way; but there was no way back this time around.

My stay proved to be uneventful in the main, although the tension within me continued to build. Reality, such as it was, and the future was dependent on the next few days. Under the circumstances, the days of my visit were relatively peaceful although the sleep situation continued to plague me. After a couple of days I walked the few steps to the phone box to find my fate. The voice on the other end was much more upbeat than it had been, the signs were good. With a great deal of relief on both sides, I found that I had managed to get the 2:1 that I'd missed the year before. It was no First, but that mattered not any more. I was through with something to show for the three years that were about to disappear over a backward horizon, and whatever happened in the future, I would always have the result and the degree to hold on to. I had no idea when or if it would come into use, but it was there. It was also very clear to me that it would be a long time before that point arrived. I had many more immediate problems to deal with.

A Pillar of Impotence

As my stay came to an end, I headed off to go and pick Rachel up on a Sunday afternoon. What would happen in the next few days was unpredictable, but would have a huge bearing on the future. It was a chance to maybe clear things up and at least try to get some answers and move on. The journey was much easier than it had been on the way, and was pervaded by an unexpectedly calm atmosphere. A great deal of Marley was played along the way, and we broke the journey for food at an almost deserted Lakeside; a vast contrast from those few days before. We stopped at the house on arrival as it started to rain lightly; rain on a bright summer's evening, rainbow conditions.

"I love the rain" she said, as we stepped out and began the walk to where we were to stay. Parking would prove to be a problem as it always was in Cambridge. At the house, I could park off the street, saving the ever dwindling contents of my bank account just a little. Such details meant nothing to me but had to be done as I knew what a struggle it would be over the summer, both mentally and fiscally.

Staying with friends proved to be less than ideal. The inevitable question of whether we wanted to sleep together arose immediately. There were the social niceties to be used, getting to know others, but they proved to be good hosts. It also proved to be very hard to sit down and talk.

We spent the days meandering our way around Cambridge, the obvious parts, and the places I went for peace. The veil that had hung for the past year was partially lifted and the atmosphere between us warm and friendly. We seemed to get back to where we had been when it had all started, but without being together. We spent a warm afternoon walking up from Grassy to the Lock, basking in the sunshine for a while in a silence sometimes interrupted by comment. It was never a silence where we knew not what to say, just a time when we were together, alone with our respective thoughts. Perhaps we were both merely contemplating the coming moment when we needed to talk for real, that time would come soon enough. Together, we just enjoyed the moment in our own ways. She was in my place of peace, and feeling why I spent so much time there. I was with her and calm, a calm that had become so rare in the previous year.

I took her to Grantchester, another of my peaceful sites; it greatly appealed to her religious nature as we sat in the silence of the churchyard and continued our quiet contemplations. The Sanctity of the place stayed with her for a long time in that religious but famous place; it was to be the only place where we met on religious terms for it was the only place that such things had been real to me. Tranquillity reined both physically and emotionally for us as time ticked by for the inevitable parting of our ways; she back to Sussex and me to Graduation and whatever was in stall for me after that. Her visit was to be one of the last calm times for many years. We were drawn together in a different way from before, and slowly the hurt was receding as the veil went back and we set up to finally talk.

Whilst the days were spent in quiet contemplation and a slow rebuilding of our relationship in a new fashion, the nights were reserved for the usual revelry that I afforded to all my guests. Good food, drink and smoking were the fair in my favourite haunts. How could I not take her to Charlie's, that staple of my time there? I'd spent so much money there over the three years that even in this time of dire financial problems, what were a few more bills for me? Then there was Sala Thong, the Anchor, the Wrestlers, the Hat and Feathers, and the Granta; I had to show her my places to set up the future. These were all the places that had been ever present for me but would within the week become a thing of the past. It was the final death throws of the best time of my life, and I was there with the one person who meant so much more than anyone else. This time, though it was together almost by proxy, together but not together, that was how it would be from now on. At least though, we were rebuilding; for so long it seemed that that would never come about.

We finally sat down to talk on the banks of the Cam near the Fort St George on the sunny morning of her final day. I was able to release the pain of the last year and tell the one that really mattered and was the key to what had happened exactly how badly life had gone wrong. She never lifted the veil enough to tell me why or anything of what went wrong on her part, but the bond was rekindled. She was alarmed but so caring as the impact became apparent to her. The silence of the last few days had gone to be replaced by at least the start of where we went from here. We were interrupted by a passing vagrant who amusingly suggested to us that perhaps we should get together, but never said what made him say that. Had there been any tension that would surely have dispelled it, but we were now back into the comfort of how we used to be; for a brief few moments, we were both in at peace in our respective if different ways. But we also both knew that within hours we would have to part in different directions, a prospect that neither of us relished. Our time was to be so brief but there was nothing we could do; life had to go on, hers in Sussex, and mine in college and my final appointment at Cambridge.

It was in the early afternoon that I drove her in silence to the station. We listened to Paul Simon as the peace of that morning began to fall apart; neither of wanted this parting. As we waited we talked quietly, both holding the tears back from one another. With an embrace and a wave she was gone. We were now both alone, her on a train, and me in the car as I headed back out to Grassy. We had agreed to meet in the summer as she returned holiday close to my home; something to look forward to, but for now I had to deal with my rapidly collapsing mental state. As I got there, the tears erupted behind the ever present dark glasses which for once were justified by the strong glare of the summer sun. Boats and people passed me by as I walked, all oblivious to their intrusion into my pain, and to the pain itself. I had one more night to stay with my friends who would be out for their Graduation dinner, then my final night in the house. Unable to be alone but unable to turn to anyone, I resolved to get as drunk as possible, that was the only way to get through such a night of pain. It proved to be the night that my life changed and I took a step closer to breakdown.

As I aimlessly wandered the streets of Cambridge for the rest of the afternoon, I tried desperately to bring some stability to the mental turmoil that had ensued. That peace of the morning had gone to be replaced by a kind of mental freefall the like of which I had never experienced before; my sanity was collapsing into a messy heap. Having eaten a little, I headed out from Lensfield Road to the Granta to sit by the riverside and drink myself into a stupor. I settled with a pint of Stella, then another, and then another. The stream of alcohol took over my ability to count as I was alone with my racing thoughts and Rachel's voice. The voice and stream of thought cascaded together, each individual process taken over by the next like the acoustics of Sacre Coeur, so massive that each passing thought blotted out the present and then reversed in on itself. I was oblivious to all around except on the regular trips to the bar, just overtaken by my own anguish.

Then out of the chaos, an amazing clarity appeared. A light, a beacon, a lantern in the darkness. The solution emerged as if it had been there all the time but I had just failed to see it, or not been able to accept it. Kill yourself. The thought flashed across my consciousness. The thought had been the terrible backdrop to the last year, one that I could never allow myself to think about actively. Now it was the only way forward. I lived in total mental darkness, now here the light leading the way was emerging. From darkness came a new light, but it was one that was veiled and cloaked in a greater darkness than was there already. But it was totally clear what I had to do from now on. Everything would head in that direction now, overriding all other thoughts.

This revelation was not clear to anyone there all at, I was the most enlightened of those customers. My demeanour continued as just someone sitting alone in a pub getting quietly drunk. To me, it was like finding God or the answer to all things; I was now totally clear and in command of my faculties, from chaos had come order. Now all I needed to do was work out the best way to achieve this strange goal. It was like a line in the sand which I had wanted to cross for some time, and I was now ready to take, and indeed had taken the step across; my mental Rubicon was now crossed. I knew I'd have to bide my time, but at least for the first time in over a year the path to the future was now illuminated. It never occurred to me that this course was so anathema to those around me. This was just the norm now, wisdom at last.

As the pub closed, I somehow managed to make my way back to Lensfield Road in my drunkenness, and settled for a long, and for once, undisturbed sleep. I slept so well I missed an ambulance arriving in the middle of the night attending to a domestic incident where I was staying. I was now completely shut off from the world around. Oblivion would get closer by the day from now on.

My return to the house the following afternoon was a time of mixed emotions. It was quiet and empty on my return, just as it had been at the end of the Easter term when I'd vainly tried to bring some semblance of a future from the rapidly disintegrating present. It had been such a place of refuge for that final year, a place of great joy, yet a place that had witnessed such desolation as had become of my life. I reflected on the great parties and breakfasts we had had there, of the fight for the two bathrooms, and of the snowball fights with the kids from across the road. There had been the clichéd idea that in eight years I had only progressed to over the road. I enjoyed the solitude and despair in equal measure as I prepared for the final night in the place that had been my home through the trauma. I had my sense of purpose now, the mission of the previous night still burning strong on my conscious. And then there was tomorrow to get through, the official end of it all.

I must finish my thoughts. Got to get them done before the others get back. This is mine and no one must interfere. They keep intruding into your space. There was a wave of determination to complete my inane ramblings that I'd started before. There was a need to complete business before it was too late. Must get it done. They can't interfere. For but a little while, these thoughts overcame the constant thoughts of Rachel and her echoing voice. The end was in sight but I had to get my affairs in order before it was too late. It seemed better to get it done here where I felt comfortable rather than back in Kent where the interruptions would be too great. I settled down for a while in the silence to bring some sort of end to it all, get my final reflections there in my book. I didn't really know why I was doing it or what would happen to it, but it seemed the most important thing to do at the time.

When I'd finished I was overtaken by sadness at where it had all gone to. There was also a great deal of dread for the morrow, the ceremony that was to come and the fact that they would be there. We were only allowed two people to come to the Senate House, and though it was last thing I wanted, I had had to agree that my mother should come along with my sister. And I knew that there would be the inevitable wallowing in the occasion by the former. I had no desire to have it recorded in any way but knew there would be a fight to get photos taken. I also knew that she would try to hijack the occasion just as she had done at my sister's Graduation three years before. In theory it was my day; in reality, I knew it would be different.

The others arrived back late in the afternoon. I was not alone in my fears for the future. Few had a great deal of hope for the future as the recession had hit so hard. There was an all around feeling of despondency but people tried to make light of the situation. No one had any inkling of the now out of control workings of my mind. Although they knew of Rachel, they had no real idea of what effect she had had on me. While others pondered on the vagaries of the job market, I was in the trying to get through the day mode. Her parting words kept running in circles around my mind; "I'm so sorry", "I'm so sorry" over and over again. But whatever our respective circumstances, whether it was to employment, a course, unemployment, or catastrophic breakdown, we were planning on going out in the same way that we had lived for the last three years. There was time for one last in house party to be had. Even with the bleakness of the situation, that had to be done. I joined in as ever letting the alcohol try to dampen the pain as much as I could. I was unable to blot Rachel out however much I drank. As it finally ended in all ways, I slept badly in my room for the last time.

Cambridge Colleges graduate in age order, excepting the two Royal Colleges which go first over a period of two days. Being from a Nineteenth Century College, we were due to process to the Senate House in mid afternoon on the Saturday. Dressed in our fine regalia with Ermine hoods, each group of students was led to the Senate House at the prescribed time, stopping all the traffic in their wake. Such was the perceived significance of the University in the city, such disruption was not only allowed but to be expected. Prior to our turn to take part in the archaic ceremony there was a lunch in the Hall for all graduates and their guests. All dressed for the occasion, I went to the lunch with mother and sister in tow, and in a great deal of mental discomfort. It was very hot and crowded as we all prepared for the end; families throughout revelled in the achievements of their respective offspring, whilst we wilted in our over dressed state.

Towards the end of lunch, I began to feel a series of unfamiliar sensations. I started to burn up in the heat. Dizziness came over me, and pins and needles started to overtake my whole body. Waves of panic came over me. There was a desperate need for nicotine. What the fuck is happening? Get out. I've got to get out of here. My thoughts raced away from me, but I maintained the survival need to keep this to myself. Making some inane excuse that I had to get some air, I virtually fled the hall. All over I seemed to be seizing up. I had no idea what was going on. People seemed to be moving in all directions, and the noise of those lunching grew in some kind of wild crescendo. I can't cope! For fuck's sake someone please help me! My capacity to move my limbs lessened as I headed for the exit. Am I going to make it out of here? I've got to get out! Where shall I go? There's nowhere to hide! All around me, people blithely continued to enjoy their lunch. Time slowed down with each step.

I reached the outside door after what seemed an eternal race, but a race from what? I had no idea what was going on. All I knew was that I'd had to get out of there. Now that I was out, there was the what next question to deal with. Unable to walk any further and lost as to what to do, I sat on the steps outside breathing heavily. With some effort to move my arms I pulled out and lit a cigarette. Inhaling in rapid bursts, the panic slowly began to subside. The pins and needles dissipated, and the breathing got slower. One cigarette, another, and then another. Calm was restored but I was in a state of shock as to what had happened. The panic was gone but I was at a loss as to how to explain it. After what was probably just a few minutes, I returned to lunch and the family. Back to pretending that all was alright and looking forward to the ceremony. Back to living the lies that would be the future, and had indeed been the past for as long as I could remember. This was to be the first of many panic attacks that were to cripple my capacity to function for a long time to come. They eventually became so frequent and alarming that I spent years avoiding anywhere where they were likely to occur. Crowds became one of my greatest fears as time moved on.

Having finished lunch we processed to the Senate House in a long column four across. The ceremony itself smacked of some ancient act of suzerainty to some great Lord or King. We held the finger of the Praelector as we were presented. We knelt, hands clasped as if in prayer. Hats were doffed with some regularity, and a great deal of incomprehensible Latin was spoken. With a bow after each of our turns, we each turned away and left the building. People stood with champagne as they awaited their friends and offspring. Finally it was over.

There was the expected argument over photos to which I reluctantly agreed. In the last few hours, all I wanted was to have a final farewell with my peers. Of course I didn't get it. It was to be all about the family just as I'd anticipated. Nothing had been arranged for the post ceremony period so we all retired to a family home in Cambridge. Champagne and smoked salmon sandwiches were the order of the day on that warm afternoon. We played croquet as the late afternoon set in late in June. This was to be our final Cambridge farewell for real. We would all meet up for Henley the following week, but it would be under very different circumstances then; life and its pitfalls would be much more real then. It would only be Henley that was false then. We were all now entitled to put the letters BA after our names. Four years from then it would be upgraded to MA (Cantab); the pretension carried on for life.

We stayed with my sister that night just a few miles out of Cambridge. The following day was to be Miriam's 24th birthday. We were to have what my parents would have regarded as a nice family birthday, where we were all together for a special occasion. In fact neither Miriam nor myself, nor indeed my brother in law wanted such an occasion. It was just another example of the illusion that they regarded as our family. Everything was based on bullshit. In the afternoon, I made my excuses of needing to go for a walk and left. I sat alone in the sun in the carnage of the building site that backed onto Miriam's house. There was desolation all around but a great sense of calm. I watched the butterflies peacefully flitter about. I was completely enclosed in my world, alone but for Rachel. The thinking and her voice went on in the quiet. The first thoughts of how to take the suicide plan to fruition started to form in my head. I knew it was coming but I also knew that I had to get it right, and with the least amount of pain. I returned after what seemed an age to the house for birthday cake. It was, as ever when my mother was involved, an entirely sober night. An almost total lack of sleep the night before would be the start of things to come. Without a drink there was almost no chance of sleep that night, and so it transpired.

The next evening, I started the long drive back to Kent. There was more of a car park on the M11 than on the M25, but at least it delayed the inevitable arrival. I knew I was headed for the oblivion of suicide, but I had to get through the extreme pain and nothingness of the family home first. That dread hung heavily over me as I travelled. Life was over, I just had to endure a few more weeks before the finish; and I had to endure it cut off from anyone I wanted to see, and in the atmosphere of a war zone. "Home" had always been a war zone. I'd endured it all my life, but until the illness struck I had managed to deal with it. After that point, I had been the focus of that strange maternal venom that was the norm for us. I'd promised myself the previous summer that I would never return to that hell, but I was now far too ill to prevent it. My last few weeks would be lived mainly in a cauldron of hate. There would be escapes along the way, but from now on these would always be temporary. Cambridge had always been my home, but that was gone too. The only escape now was death; and death would have to wait.

Chapter 7

Sion Deserta

That first night back in Kent I slipped out of the house in the early hours, got in the car and simply drove without any particular aim or destination in mind. I had tried to sleep but that had failed miserably so I just decided to get out for a while. With a tape on and an eternal chain of cigarettes, I found myself in Dover. For the next few hours I wandered the largely deserted streets in my own world. From time to time I stopped and sat down on a passing bench and reflected. The occasional pedestrian came by, I got a strange look from two passing policemen, but was generally alone and oblivious, with just my thoughts and Rachel racing in my head. There was an ever pervading sense of loneliness and isolation as I tried to come to grips with the situation that I now had to face. Everything that mattered had gone with only the fleeting chance of getting any of it back. Life had become a deserted place; all those possibilities were now just a memory that had passed into my past.

Through my nocturnal wanders, I was unaware of any possible dangers that lurked in the darkness. Those passing were merely people who were intruding into my world in a peripheral way. Effectively, I was shut down from any form of reality. As the first signs of the dawn appeared in the east I decided to go back and try to get some sleep. It seemed vital that no one should know of my travels, and that no one should be woken. I drove back through blinding fog, went in and slipped quietly under the covers as the day became lighter. Then after such a short space of time came the call, "it's 8 o' clock, time to get up". This set the pattern for the future, this was the way we live a normal life, and normal people get up at that time and have a normal family breakfast. Each night I struggled to sleep until it was beginning to get light, and each morning came that same call, day in day out. Just as each day started like that, so each night started with me slipping out late and going to the car. Often I would just sit there rather than travel, with just my thoughts, my music, my cigarettes, and her voice.

To add to the problems that I faced, the harsh financial reality of graduating struck almost immediately. I went along to sign on at the local DHSS office straight away. Having filled in the relevant forms, they hastily arranged an interview to look at my situation. Having explained that I had just graduated, I was informed that they would give me a week to find a real job and after that, I would have to take anything on offer. The ethos was simply to get as many people off the books as fast as possible just to make the figures look better and hide the recession that was staring so many people in the face. The fact that there were no jobs about seemed to be irrelevant, as well as the fact that I had spent so many years of being primed that education was the key to getting on in the future. I was refused money to which I was entitled because they claimed I hadn't been "actively seeking work" in the last couple of weeks of Cambridge.

I was required to appear at a prescribed time every to two weeks to sign on the line. In addition, they would recall me in the future at various stages for another interview at which I had to bring proof of what I had done to get work. The amount paid was pitifully low; after paying the bare minimum essentials of food, I was left with the grand total of £19 per week on which to live. In their terms, the law had spoken and I was financially fucked for however long it took to get a job, any job. I also knew full well that with my mental deterioration, there was absolutely no chance of me able to work even if I could get a job.

That situation was bad enough but it got worse very quickly. Having had money and overdrafts shoved in my face for the three years of my course, graduation brought a swift response from the bank. Within a week of graduation, they were on to me about paying off my overdraft. The figures were small and I wasn't even at or over the limit, but they wanted it back straight away. As my branch was in Cambridge, I decided to transfer it to Kent to make it easier to deal with. I went in to speak to them and was asked if I had a job. When I replied that I didn't, I was told that I'd have to pay it off, close the account, and then start a new one. With an attitude like that, I speculated to myself about how stupid they were if they thought I was likely to open another account with them after that. I was reduced to borrowing from my parents and waiting for the money I was owed by the Football Club to arrive. I hated having to borrow from them as it was one more tie and source of conflict for me to deal with. But I had little choice; it was just replacing one problem with another.

Despite the financial problems, I made it to Henley to meet up with the others the following week. The decadence of Henley made our life in Cambridge look positively unpretentious; the life we had just left seemed so real in comparison. I had set off in blazer and tie in my battered yellow VW around the M25 to pick some people up in north London, then on anti clockwise towards Henley. One of my house mates had been rowing that week but they had been knocked out of their competition. They had been put up for the week in a family home on the edge of the town, and it had been arranged that the supporters could camp there and leave their cars. Having dumped the car, we headed for the river. It was strikingly clear that this was purely a social occasion for most of the packed crowd, very few of whom seemed to have any idea about rowing. Pimm's and champagne flowed in equal measure at vast expense; the former was selling at £7 a pint but no one seemed to care. Having decided that camping was an idea I could do without, and having a bed on offer in Ascot, I stayed sober and drove off after an exhausting day. Amid the pretension, the mental mayhem was temporarily put aside, and for a rare night, I slept well.

It proved to be only a temporary respite. The following day we went back and somehow managed to get into the Steward's enclosure for even more decadence. I met friends from school there, but it could not stop the mental free fall. I started to connect the falseness of the surroundings with the idea that I was a fraud and that I should never have been there. Enclosed by wealth and the trappings thereof, despair closed me in all around. What the fuck are you doing here? You don't deserve to be here. You're a fake and fraud. Get back to your miserable little life. The thoughts kept colliding as I shut off from all that was around. We left late in the afternoon for Matt's house. I followed my other house mate through the traffic chaos of the end of the regatta, and after a very stressful journey arrived just about ready to drop.

That night we ate, drank and swam in the pool. It was like the old days but we all knew that that was finished. The girl from Ohio was there. She was due to fly home within a few days, and, as before, kept up the pressure on me. That was way beyond what I could cope with, and once again I had to spurn her. She wanted me to come to the airport to see her off, but I simply couldn't afford the petrol. As we all parted the next morning, I headed for oblivion and she headed back to the States. I never saw her again, but within a couple of months she was to have a profound effect on my life in an unexpected way.

The days between trips took on an air of eternal drift. Each passed so slowly as I tried to wipe away the hours. Although I saw no one of note between times, I endeavoured to get out of the house as much as possible. Many hours were spent aimlessly wandering the streets, sitting by the sea, and hidden amongst the reeds by the canal. Each of these journeys took me further and further from anything that was real. Reality was reduced to coming out of my room for meals, leaving the house for no particular purpose other than to try to alleviate the building pressure. Whatever I did and wherever I went, the quiet contemplations continued, its pace increasing as each day drifted by. When indoors, I blankly stared at the TV screen in an uncomprehending way. When I could follow what was on, I became obsessed with closing music of programmes and their credits; each represented another hour or part hour gone, but also the end of any distraction. Very quickly I began to turn off the end of things, or to hit the mute button just to get by the ensuing pain. As each day finally drew to a close, I tried desperately to get some sleep before the inevitable and ridiculous call to the day; but each attempt always ended fruitlessly, the sleep being so short and interrupted that it felt it had never taken place.

After a few weeks of this, I finally resolved to see a Doctor just to try to get some sleeping pills or something to help. For a long time I had known that sooner or later I would have to go down that course although I had serious doubts that anything they could do would help. I also knew that they would probably tell me it was more serious than just sleeplessness. Still registered in Cambridge, I went to my old surgery to fill in the relevant paper work to be seen as a visitor, not really knowing that this would be the first of hundreds of time that I would have to fill something in for the NHS or the DHSS. After all, I'd be dead soon so I'd ceased to think in anything but the very shortest of terms. My old Doctor was on holiday so I went in to see an unfamiliar face. We talked for a while, but he seemed vague and non committal. He said nothing about what he thought was wrong with me but gave me some pills "to help you sleep" and told me to come back in a week. Armed with a prescription and very little else, I headed to the chemist for collection. They gave me a bottle of small yellow pills with no explanation of what they were; a week's supply of an unknown substance that I assumed was some form of sleeping tablet. That night I took the prescribed pill, and perhaps more in hope than anything else, I managed to sleep a little better. The night after that I reverted to type. For reasons I did not understand, my mother insisted on doling them out to me in case I accidentally took more than I meant to; it was like being back with the old school matron at the medicine cupboard, a memory I detested.

Increasingly my active and conscious mind turned to how I was to carry out the task in hand, vital as it was. As attractive as it seemed being so instantaneous, I rejected the idea of walking across the motorway, that would affect whoever was driving too much. Hanging sounded too painful, pills were out as I didn't think I had enough and access was limited. Each of the many options had its drawbacks and so eventually I resolved that using the car exhaust was the best bet, and it seemed safer to do it in the garage as there was less chance of being found and someone fucking it all up for me. The intention was so overwhelming that it was worked in detail, but in naive detail. The main drawback was getting access to the garage to use this method. They were going away in September so I would have to wait until then, play a waiting game. Each day became part of the countdown to the final act that would end the pain for good. The days and nights of thought increasingly revolved around this time table, but there was a great deal of time until September, especially with each twenty four hour cycle being seemingly so long and drawn out. The excruciating pain increased by the day, but had to be endured.

The following week I returned to the Doctor as requested. I was back on familiar ground with someone I knew, if not very well. It was an altogether warmer and friendlier meeting than at the previous search for help. But it was just as unenlightening a meeting as before. More questions, but still no answers. The pills were having little or no impact but I was to carry on with them for another week and then return, just as before. He asked me if I wanted to see the Mental Health Team. Feeling I had nothing to lose I agreed. I was unaware of the growing concern of the physician; in subsequent years I came to realise that the speed with which the referral was made was highly unusual. An appointment was made within days. As I left I pondered on what on earth a shrink would make of me, a thought that had been in my head for some time.

July was drifting towards its close and I was no more aware of what was going on than I had been on my return. There was no word from Rachel which began to alarm me. She would be returning near me within a week or so but I had no idea why she hadn't been in touch to arrange to meet as promised. Thoughts of her became stronger and more aggressive with each passing day. At around this time I set out on a warm afternoon to walk to nowhere in particular. As I passed close to a fallen tree trunk in the middle of a field, I felt a sudden and intense pain in my head. It was a pain the like of which I had never felt. All I could was lie down on the trunk, chain smoking, and crying out in the hope that the pain would stop. After a while I continued on my journey to nowhere just trying to blot it out but it refused to go. On my return, I tried every form of pain relief I knew but to no avail. It continued into the night further complicating the nocturnal problems. The moment that I woke it was there again. And again the next morning, and then again. It became the physical incarnation of the mental suffering. It never left in a waking moment, and became my constant companion for years to come. I was now falling to pieces both mentally and physically. I went to see the Mental Health Team on a bakingly hot and oppressive afternoon. As ever my parents insisted that they must come too, always wanting to know what was happening. We sat in a small, airless waiting room for what seemed an age. I was called into an even smaller room by a bearded man whom I took to be a psychiatrist, and a heavily accented woman whom it transpired was social worker. That was about all the sense I could make of her so strong was her accent. Then the questions started. Did I get this? Did I feel that? Was I obsessive? Each question elicited a clearly thought out if rather bemused answer.

"Do you hear voices?"
"No."

It was not until I'd spoken to others who had that I began to realise about Rachel; it was not, at that stage, a concept that I understood, and no connection was made with the questioning.

"Have you ever felt suicidal?"
"No" was my emphatic and instant response.

My mind went into instant overdrive. They mustn't know. They can't stop me. They won't stop me. Thoughts kept rushing at me, but above all I had to protect the plan now well formulated in my head.

The bearded man went on with his questioning but I was now in auto answer mode and they just passed me by, although the answers were just as coherent as before.

"The pills you have been given aren't sleeping pills" he went on, "they are anti-depressants. I think you have depression."

His statement was so bland but had a great resonance within me. So there is something wrong with me. It does exist. I'm not imagining things. There was an enormous sense of relief at that, but it was tarnished by the feeling I had of betrayal by the Doctors. Why didn't they tell? I had no answer to that thought.

He wanted to see me again in a couple of weeks and an appointment was made before they barged in with their oar. I had no desire for them to talk to them but at least it might shelve the questioning. I had no idea what the pair said to them, and they had no idea what was said to me. They got just the bare minimum as we headed back in the still sweltering heat of that late afternoon.

The summer continued on its inexorable march towards autumn and meandered into August. The physical and mental effects of the illness were now extracting a heavy toll. There had been little to break the cycle since Henley, and the isolation was almost complete. I went through each day without seeing anyone, and those I saw in passing were just intruding into my pain. The mood was lifted briefly when I had a call from an old friend inviting me over for a week or two whilst her family was on holiday. At last there was a way out, however temporary it might be. Although I knew that it would not do a great deal to stop the confusion as that would go with me, but at least I would be out of the stifling atmosphere of the house.

A Pillar of Impotence

On my next visit to the Doctor, a longer prescription was written out to cover my time away. I collected the bottle with ninety of the little yellow pills in it, the ones with the chalky texture created as they collided and rubbed against each other in transit. When I got in, I put them down next to my bed and simply left them there until it was time to go to Sussex.

Despite the potential respite, August brought a marked deterioration in my condition. Each day and night I became more desperate and moved closer to the edge. The music I listened to in my nightly forays to the car began to happen automatically in my head. In my wanderings I became accompanied by a sort of Jukebox blasting things out in my mind. There was no need to take a Walkman anywhere, it just happened anyway whether I wanted it or not. Places, music and thoughts took on even greater symbolism. My aversion to TV music became stronger. Time was passed hour by hour not from day to day. Each day merged into the next and the respite was still too far off. The lack of news from Rachel seriously disturbed me. She had promised to meet up but seemed to have broken that promise. Maybe I had deluded myself that things were better when we had met back in Cambridge. More and more she was on my mind and in my head.

A few days before I was due to head off to see Becky, I slipped out into the night and headed for the car. With obsessive care I silently went out of the door, down the steps and across the road to the car. It was parked under a neighbour's tree, safer off the road, but covered in a thick sticky film deposited from above. I unlocked the door and climbed in. I turned on the tape and lit a cigarette. My mind was racing and Rachel's voice was everywhere. My head throbbed and I yearned for sleep and rest. Another cigarette, then another, then the tears. She's betrayed me. Where is she? She promised. She should have been back by now. Thoughts echoed around my head, interspersed with her. My thoughtful questions were never answered by her although I knew from experience that she never did answer me, but just kept on talking. I was craving the arrival of September and the final planned release. Release in the car in which I was sitting. It was all I had left in the world, and it was mine.

It was a night that on the face of it was no different from all the others that summer. But it was different, for on this particular night, I finally cracked. Use the pills! The final thought of clarity.

Chapter 8

Passus et Sepultus Est

He stood at the end of the bed in a long white coat. He was middle-aged and tall. Around him stood a group of others, similarly coated but much younger. Through the haze that was my consciousness I gradually became aware of what he was and what he was doing. A torrent of abuse belched from his mouth and was lapped up by his minions. The consultant playing to his audience, those who knew no better, and hung on his every insult. He seemed to think that telling me how stupid I was and how I'd wasted so much of their valuable time and resources would be of some benefit. The more aware and awake I became the more the rage crescendoed in my mind.

I lay in bed barely able to move and unable to speak in more than a hoarse whisper. His words kept coming. My mind went back into overdrive. Filled with hate and out of control I was trapped. Fuck off you fucking cunt. Where the fuck do you get off telling me this? I didn't want to live. Nobody asked you to save me. I want to fucking kill you. The thoughts flew out in torrents. Yet they were tempered by my usual self composure. You can't say that to him. He doesn't know what he is saying. Be still and stay quiet. It will pass.

But it didn't pass. I fought to overcome the thoughts. My hooded eyes focused on one of his audience. A young, dark skinned, rather plump man stood by his side. His face had a kind of knowing grin on it. He was desperate to learn from the master. He looks like a pig. A faint thought followed immediately by another about whether it was racist to think that or not. But it wasn't about the colour of his skin, he just looked like a pig. If you focus on the pig, maybe you can blot it out. He's a pig. He's a pig. The thought came repetitively through my head. The arsehole's words began to wash over me and gradually disappeared. My eyes flicked over his acolytes. What fools they all were. This was indoctrination into the sacred world of the physician; save life whatever the consequences. Nobody seemed to give a shit about what those consequences were for me, I was just there taking up a bed and wasting their time. I was back from the dead physically, but dead and buried mentally. I'd survived and nothing had changed.

My stay in hospital was both vague and clear. Small incidents of extreme clarity interspersed with periods of complete blackout. Time and the days had no meaning there, and I had no idea when I woke how long I had been there, or how long I was to stay. I was only vaguely aware of night and day, light and dark, heat and cold was just accompaniments to the drift. People came in and out to see me, but I was often unaware that they had been or what they had done. Consciousness was just a passing phase for me, as it came and left with no particular pattern to it.

When I first became aware of the unfortunate bout of survival, I was eating a curry for lunch. I must have been eating in an unaware way as I looked down to see myself covered in the contents of plate all down my front. The awareness struck suddenly half way through, as if I'd sleep walked into where I seemed to be and jolted awake. There was no thought of the failures of survival, no lights at the end of a tunnel, no God or any of the things people apparently see when they have a near death experience. Through some internal instinct I knew without thinking that it had been a very close brush with death. To my mind it was clearly not close enough.

My throat was severely constricted, and I found it extremely hard to even try to swallow let alone succeed. That situation, combined with a chronic shakiness that I had picked up, put paid to my lunch. The food I did manage to get into my mouth tasted very good, but I was unable to correlate it with everyone's belief about hospital food. Sitting next to the bed were my parents. I tried to speak but little came out above a rough whisper.

"I like it, but I can't eat it." I had to repeat this short statement several times before it became comprehensible to them. I had no feeling of wanting to see them, or not wanting to see them; they were just there.

It was hot in there, and it was only the fact that it was light and I was eating that I was able to ascertain that it must be the afternoon. I glanced around the room to try and find some bearings as to where I was. I was in the bed nearest to the corridor in the bay of a ward. There were six beds in there, one of which was empty. I was struck by the age of those around me, unaware that they were struck by my age more than me of theirs. There was man in the corner who was intently watching a small TV while he was eating his lunch. The other three there were much older than him or I.

In what seemed like the blink of an eye, I fell back into the unconsciousness from whence I had come. So started my stay there, long periods of welcome oblivion interspersed by such incidents. Some were welcome, others were horrific. The next time that I was aware of being awake, the bed opposite had been filled, and the ward was up to its capacity. He was an old man who looked very ill. He often had the oxygen mask from above the bed over his face, and he had a huge dressing over some abdominal wound. I mused on what that mask was like but I never used it.

The first morning I remember at the hospital, a middle-aged man came around the small ward with a trolley laden with food, drinks and newspapers. I had a vague thought that I wanted a newspaper to at least try to read. Then it dawned on me that I had no money to buy one with. Vaguely disappointed I must have dropped off again and he drifted from my thoughts. Later I awoke again to find my parents there. I mentioned the newspaper incident to them and was greeted by a bemused look on their faces. They told me that they'd left some money for me in my wash bag. I was not even aware that there was such a thing in my possession, let alone that it contained money. The thought of getting up beyond the bed was still alien to me. In their own inimitable way, they clung to the idea that the intricacies of normality, however mundane they were, were not on the agenda in there. Then I must have passed out again.

My eyes slid open again. Miriam was sitting close to the bed. For the first time since that night my mind went into overdrive. What's she doing here? She should be at work. Why would she want to see me? I couldn't understand at all why she was there, and why she would bother to take time off to be there. Lost and confused I surveyed her face; it seemed so sad and upset, but this just added to my confusion. Whatever she said never made it through to my understanding mind, just more words directed at me that failed to penetrate beyond my nearly closed eyes. For the whole time she was down she never made an impact apart from being there on that day. It was many years before I realised that she was a witness to the next part of this strange journey that was being planned and led by others. I no longer had any control over what was happening.

Slowly with the passing hours, I began to glean more of what had happened; no one told me anything directly, it was just little bits of the puzzle that slipped from people's mouths as they struggled inanely for what to say to me. It seemed I had been in a coma for a number of days; that number was never specified. My breathing had stopped a couple of times in the ambulance. I'd been kept in the rather curiously named "Intensive Therapy Unit". I was in Cambridge Ward which everyone seemed to think I would like. They hadn't known precisely what I had taken; no one knew that I even had painkillers so they had no idea of the quantity taken. I'd spent some time on a ventilator. The hardest part to deal with was finding out how I had been found. By one of the bizarre twists of fate that seem to litter people's lives, my parents had bumped into a retired Doctor friend whilst swimming in the sea early in the morning. As chance would have it, they invited him back for coffee that day, and, when the 8 o' clock call had come and failed to wake me, he realised what had happened and hastened the ambulance. On hearing this, a great enmity arose on my part concerning him. Maybe he was the one who should take the blame for this unfortunate story of survival. I never really forgave him for that. Another Doctor playing God with my life; he was the first of many. So the little quirks of life that are chance and coincidence had played their part; more things beyond my control.

Over time my periods of consciousness increased but so did the questions. More people dropped in to see me, but the inevitable recriminations, and the desire for answers became stronger. The others in the bay wanted to know why I was there; "what is wrong with you?" became an ever increasing question. It never struck me as odd that someone as young as me was there, but it seemed to have a great resonance for those around. The constriction to my throat and its related handicap on my speech began to ease. I mused on the idea of seeing one of my musical friends who lived close by. But much as I wanted to see her, I knew that the start of the explanations would have to come, and I wasn't ready to face that. It was one thing in a group of strangers that I was never likely to see again, but to people who knew me it was a much harder prospect; sadly I was forced to reject that notion.

A Pillar of Impotence

She sat on the chair by the bed as I emerged once again from my drug induced slumbers. She sat quietly, reading her book, unaware that I was awake. She was a young nurse with long blonde hair and a friendly face. I wondered why she was there; another attack from the medical profession or just someone sent to be with me. As I stirred she started to talk to me. There was sadness in her face and in her voice as she tried hard to understand where I was coming from. She spoke quietly but with great compassion, someone who wanted to help.

"You're so young" she said, "why did you do it when you have so much to live for?"

"I've done more in my time than most people do in their lifetimes" was my reply. Whether that was a sign of vanity, arrogance, delusion or madness I don't know, but that was my mindset. I told her of Rachel and the other catastrophes that had blighted my life, but although she couldn't comprehend my actions, the friendliness never wavered. Though shocked she gave little away. It was so different from the cunt in the white coat who had been my only other contact with the profession, at least in my awareness. When I awoke next she was gone. I never saw her again, but the sense that at least someone cared stayed with me throughout my stay, and as time went by with no hint of getting better.

Then came the inevitable shrink. It was another stiflingly hot afternoon in the airless ward. England had just beaten the West Indies in the Test Match but I'd missed it as I was asleep. The younger man in the opposite corner told me as I woke. Still unsteady on my feet, I staggered to the toilet, and on my return I was sent off to a small room that was equally airless. A small Asian man with a balding head sat there. Then the questions started. How had I done it? Had I locked the door? Had I meant it? Who was Rachel? Had we had sex? What about Cambridge? What was I going to do for a job? As he went on and on, I answered each question in an entirely detached way. As it became obvious that I was talking to the proverbial brick wall, I became more and more irritated and uncomfortable. As was to prove the case as time went by, there were many questions but no answers. From what little I could make of his thinking, it was clear that he had no idea what I was talking about, or what it felt like to me. I just got an increasingly incredulous look from him. Having gained nothing from the meeting, I headed back with my opinion hardening against Doctors. Unlike the nurse, they all seemed to be completely devoid of compassion or understanding. It was a belief that was to be reinforced as time went by, each of those that I met seemed to be the same. Nobody seemed to give a shit about what I thought or felt, they only cared about their erroneous opinions.

It was nearly lunch time when they came to tell me I was well enough to go home. By that stage my throat and voice were almost back to normal, and, although still unsteady, I could get around much better. I was now spending more time conscious than I had been and was deemed to be well. I may have been better physically, but mentally I was getting worse again. The more time I was awake, the more Rachel came back into my being.

I got dressed and packed my stuff, marginally disappointed that I was to miss a lunch that at least I had ordered. Having said goodbye to the others in the bay and to some of the staff, we got in the car and headed home. On the journey I started to reflect on things. Nothing had changed and I had nothing to get back to. My situation was utterly unchanged from where it had been. For all the questions that had been asked, nobody had offered anything to help. No one had said what would happen next. My life was still in a complete mess, and Rachel was beginning to become active again. I reflected on what to say to people, how to deal with the unmentionable. No one who mattered knew, but it was only a matter of time before they did. I had to call Becky about going down to see her so something had to be said. And then there was my next real conversation with Rachel. How would she take it? My stay had just been an unreal interlude away from the hell that was my daily life. The people at the hospital had been doing what they perceived to be their job; saving life was the be all and end all of their professional incarnation. No thought had been given to me or the devastating effect their actions would have on me. The resentment stiffened as we headed back, back to where we had been however long ago it had been. No one even told me how long I had been there.

Back in isolation we ate lunch, all of us pondering on what would happen next. It was a quiet time, no one knowing quite what to do or say. Lost as I was, the others were too. I came down later in the afternoon to find my mum writing a thank you card to the staff. I nearly exploded in rage on the spot, but I managed to internalise the fury; back to my usual way of doing things. Seething with anger, I left the house and headed back to my usual summer haunts. For the first time in days I smoked a cigarette, and slowly things began to calm down. I had failed and nothing had changed. But far worse was about to come; the man with the beard would be over in a couple of days, and he would bring with him a different kind of hell.

Chapter 9

The Archbishop's Palace

He paced the corridor mumbling to himself. All day long he patrolled the chequered floors of the labyrinth. When approached he spoke the same words each time.

"Got a cigarette sir, got 10p?" over and over.

What he mumbled the rest of the time was not known. Rumours of his vast intelligence swept that place. No one seemed to know how long he had been there, but he kept up his sojourn day after day; what was clear though was that he was unlikely to leave that place. Each passing traveller was asked that same question, and if they responded to his request, he'd ask for another, then another.

That place, named after a long dead Saint and Archbishop, was like an eternal corridor that seemed to go on for miles, ready to swallow up those who were lost. The checks of the floor were mirrored by huge pipes overhead. Many doors led off those cloisters, where they led was unknown to most. Whether there were other sentinels I never found out, but this one was always there. They said his name was John; but we weren't even sure if that was true.

The bearded man came late on another hot and humid afternoon. We adjourned to my room, out of the way in the place that had been my cell and refuge since my return. It was small and cramped with but one chair, a bed, and a desk. He sat wearily down on the chair with another incredulous look on his face; that look was all I seemed to get from people after my unfortunate survival.

"When I spoke to you before, you said you had never felt suicidal. Why did you say that?"
"I didn't want you to stop me" was my immediate response, just as swift as when he had asked the original question.

Another bemused and slightly angry look came across his face. I could almost see the mechanisms of his mind working, asking questions to himself. It must have seemed incomprehensible to him, that I could come to him for assessment when I knew full well what was about to happen. But in my own way it was what I had had to do. I'd never held the belief that there was anything that could be done to help me, but I'd gone to see him anyway. I still remembered the relief I had felt when he had accepted that there was something wrong with me, but there was still no hope to come out of the meeting.

Yet here we were again, on slightly more familiar territory, with very little change. When waiting for him to arrive, I really had no idea what he was going to do or say. His initial question was all that I could anticipate, the rest had not entered my thinking. For me the last few days had been a disastrous set back, but the determination to die was just as strong; I merely had to find another way to get it right. But now that they were aware of my true intentions, the job would be that much harder to complete. Despite the peculiarly doubting questions of the hospital staff, he knew it was for real.

Still looking bemused by my initial response to the opening salvo, he continued to ask his questions, but they went over my head. The responses went back to the automatic pilot I took on in those days. Then came his conclusion.

"I think you need to go into hospital for a while. I've made the necessary arrangements for tomorrow."
"If you think it will help, I'll do it."

The response came before the implications of the statement had sunk in. As a child in Cambridge, we had often joked that people would be taken away in a yellow van by the men in white coats to Fulbourn. Where the yellow van came from I have no idea, but the idea was rather Dickensian. We knew the place existed, but it was just an idea of fantasy. It was just a joke, and none of us knew what the place was really like. What we did know was that it was a pretty terrifying thought, something that you would only say to children to frighten them. Now I was faced with that as a reality, but was convinced it couldn't be as bad as we thought it would be.

As a very young child, I'd seen a psychologist at his office in the grounds of an old asylum. It was the place where the funny people lived but my memories were only vague. Yet that was in the 1970s, and things had to have moved on from there; change has to come over fifteen or so years. Logic had to prevail.

My thoughts on going there were vague and confused. It seemed just a concept to me, one that I had no real idea of what it would be like. I still had some belief that it could only do me good as these people were the experts on whatever it was that was afflicting me. On the other hand, the urge to commit suicide was still overwhelming. Neither the staffs at this hospital nor the bearded man were going to stop me; it was a case of biding my time again. But I saw nothing to lose by going there.

The following morning I was in an unusually upbeat mood. The heat of the advancing summer was still there, but the oppressive humidity had been replaced by a fresher outlook. Although I had little idea of what this place would be like, the prospect of being in hospital for an indeterminate length of time in highly humid conditions did not appeal greatly. I went into town to buy a few bits and pieces before setting off for the place that was at that time unknown to me. I bought a book to keep me busy, unaware yet that my capacity to read had all but deserted me. Thinking that hospitals are sterile and clean places, I decided that I'd better not take my cigarettes. I'd survived those days in hospital without smoking at all, and painful though it might be, I'd have to survive further. More utter naivety as to what was to come, but my mind was only functioning in terms of preconceived ideas. My memories of those visits in the 70s were not recalled that day; hospitals were all the same as far as my mind would have it, and that meant not being able to smoke. It never occurred to me that it might be possible to go outside, or that there would be a smoking room on the ward.

We undertook the journey into the unknown at lunchtime. It was unknown in all senses to me, I knew not what was going to happen there, nor was I aware enough to work out where I was going. After a while, we travelled along a narrow road bordered for much of its length by boarded up houses. It seemed as if we were passing through some sort of ghost town, a long abandoned and forgotten settlement that was of no use to anyone. We turned to the right at a crossroads not far from where the houses had started; more abodes of similar ilk edged along this road too. A pub appeared on the left.

It looked sad, forlorn, and rundown. Then there was a gatehouse on the right. We swung into the road and through what must have once been grand gates. Ahead was a long drive, marked on either side by a row of impressively old trees. They disappeared into the distance, and gave the sense of guiding the travellers to the destination that could not be imagined unless it had been witnessed before. Behind the trees were a series of red brick building, increasing in size the further along the road we got. Of similar appearance to those boarded houses we'd passed earlier, these building also had the air of decay and neglect. Some of these were also abandoned; others seemed to still be in use, although they betrayed no clue as to what that use was today.

The density of red brick became continuous at the end of the long drive. The trees gave way to a large field with a cricket square roped off, but apparently little used. A decrepit pavilion stood at its corner. Opposite was a vast building of red brick. It was long but even from there clearly had great depth to it. It reminded me a great deal of my places of residence on both my stints living in Cambridge; a mid to late Victorian building of similar design but much greater scale than those in Cambridge. Towers and turrets seemed to emit from various points on the building. All had that same sheen of decay we had seen on the main road. There was a terrible majesty to this place even in the early 90s. It had clearly been an impressive sight in its early days, and although those days were long gone now, there was still an air to it. But there was also a sense of great dread and foreboding. I felt the first inklings of unease within me. I already sensed that I may have made a big mistake by agreeing to go there. If that sense was shared by the others I don't know; nothing was said by anyone that I can recall. But having completely blotted out the presence of Miriam, I cannot be sure.

The grounds were deserted, and there was no outward sign of human habitation within. There was an eerie silence as we approached a door of flexible plastic on the far left hand side of the main building. The plastic slapped together as we entered creating the only sound we had heard since our arrival. We emerged into a long and gloomy corridor. The floor was marked by a large black and white checked cover of some indeterminate substance. Above were huge pipes that disappeared into the distance as far as we could see. Finally there were signs of life in the dingy interior. An elderly man who stooped somewhat approached us shuffling down the corridor. He mumbled as he came.

"Got a cigarette sir, got 10p?"

On meeting no response, he shuffled back off into the gloom. We climbed the stairs and arrived at our destination. An enormous metal door stood before us barring the way not only in, but more alarmingly, the way out. It had a small viewing point that opened inwards. The sense of foreboding changed to a feeling of absolute dread. This is a prison. Why did I agree to come here? I must be mad. That's why I'm here! The thought process started to get out of control at that point. But I knew that there was no way out now. We pressed the rather tacky doorbell. First the shutter opened, and then the heavy door swung slowly open with a curious noise. It was very old and betrayed a terrible symbolism. Once in it was up to them to let you out again.

The moment that we entered, I was the subject of intense curiosity from all those about. The inmates were stirring to see the new arrival; the staff set about their business. Formalities were set in motion: into the office; the usual rounds of more questions; weighing and measuring; blood pressure. It went on but meant nothing to me. The only thing that caused any emotion in me was finding out that I had lost weight. That made no sense to me as my weight had always been stable and the thought of losing it during my first stay in hospital was anathema to me, it just didn't add up in my mind. After an unknown period of time the examination finished. Nothing that they had said to me had gone in or made any sense. With that it was time for them to go and leave me in this strange place. The iron door swung shut with a great clang behind them and they were gone. The sound of that door echoed in me for some time after. The symbolism was dramatic. I knew I was trapped and was getting more afraid by the second. I was a prisoner, but one who had committed no crime. We were all at the mercy of those in charge, subject to all their whims and emotions. We were entirely subjugated to their will, it was always on their say so who did, or did not go wherever. Having closed the door to the world, they retired to their office and stayed there. The pattern was set from that moment on. Now I was alone with the curious. I knew none of them.

A Pillar of Impotence

All I knew was that it was a terrible mistake coming to this place, and that I had to get out as fast as I could. But how?

The interior of this hidden world was cavernous. Essentially one long room, it was sub-divided into different areas. Immediately inside the metal portal was a small and rather make shift dining area filled with cheap and decrepit furniture, the sort you would find in a school where the budget was over stretched. There was a small kitchen that was attached, although this was kept locked most of the time. Another small room led off from there; it was empty but for a mattress on the floor. This was also locked and gave me a fearful sense, sending shivers through me just at the thought of it being there, and the realisation that I never wanted to enter it. It transpired that this was the seclusion room so I was right to be fearful. I never saw anyone put in there whilst I was at that place, one of those great feelings of relief that surely must come to all those who have been locked up. Beyond lay a vast open plan dormitory filled with aging metal beds laid out in long rows. It was just as it had been in my youth in Cambridge; the two buildings looked the same internally and externally, as if they were in a time warp. Perhaps it was just that institutions by their very nature were somewhat similar. Within this sleeping area was a small office that served as both a nursing centre and a watch tower from which control could be extended as well as the locked door and barred windows. To the right was another partition which divided off a bathroom and a TV room. All of it was wreathed in pale haze of smoke; my decision to leave my cigarettes came back to haunt me, so unprepared was I for such a place. We were all imprisoned and entombed in this grave like venue, alive only in a physical sense. This was the place of the mad and mad or not, I was there for an open-ended stay.

One by one they came to me as I sat alone and bemused in the dining area. An old man approached talking and smoking as he went. He was friendly and talked endlessly in a coherent way but so quickly did he change tack it was hard to make any sense of him. Another old man came over; he was the seer of visions. A young man with the kind of wild psychotic eyes that you see in all the Hollywood horror movies. Others were to follow later. Nobody seemed to do anything in there but smoke. My predicament was eased by their generosity and they assured me that there was a place to buy supplies, but only when they were prepared to let me out.

Late in the afternoon there was great excitement. People appeared from all over the place, and even the staff emerged from their hideaway. They opened the door of the small kitchen, pulled back the shutters and started to count heads. With great glee, it was announced to me that it was tea time, the highlight of an otherwise deathly dull afternoon. The staff didn't seem to know who was there and who wasn't. They merely counted up the number of people around and then proceeded to make the required number of cups of tea. There was no coffee allowed as it seemed that people had been known to go into the kitchen with a jar and simply fill it up with hot water from the tap. The fact that having the kitchen continuously locked except when it was tea time precluded any chance of this being done again seemed not to have crossed their minds.

A middle aged women appeared at the window and was allowed in. She was very slim, with her face so drawn her skin seemed to hang off it. She was heavily made up, in the manner of a pubescent girl who had just discovered her mother's make-up bag. She peered at me through sunken eyes.

"He's nice" was all she said. She joined us for tea and said very little, she just looked at me intently for the duration. I never found out what her name was but they told me that she was from the ward downstairs, and liked to come up for tea in the other place.

After a short while they collected in the empty cups, locked up the kitchen and disappeared back into their office. That was the extent of what was on offer there. My fears multiplied moving me closer to outright terror. It was not so much fear of those in there; that was to come later. It was the fear that I'd agreed to come here because it might help, but had made a very grave mistake. This was a loony bin in all senses of the phrase. We were just dumped there and left. There was no help there, just endless boredom, excess smoking, and no hope. Although they had no interest in those there, they still had the power to let us come and go, and we did not. It was purely up to them. Whatever was wrong with me in the first place was only going to be made worse there. I knew almost immediately that if I wasn't mad when I went in, I certainly would be if they ever let me out. But that was our lot and there was nothing to be done about it. I thought back to the old days of Fulbourn. It had just been a fantasy for us, but this was alarmingly real.

Real though it was, there was wholly unreal atmosphere to it. No one seemed to know what the truth was about the place or the people who populated it. Stories abounded, some of which made sense, and some did not. The more people I met the more I learned, or was deceived; it was just so hard to know which was which. The man who said he'd just come back from France was evasive about much but was full of warnings: do this or that, don't do this or that. Don't ever ask why they are here, and above all never show anyone your arse. He was raped by the women downstairs and wants to rape little girls. He'd tried to hang himself last week but the nurse had stopped him and beaten him up. All around were stories but were they real? Did they need to be real? Where the hell do you find any sense in any of this? Above all the overriding question in my mind was how on earth this place was ever going to help me.

Dinner came and went in the same fashion; open shutters, serve food, clear up, and fuck off back to the office. Then there was a change. I was utterly confused by all I had seen that day when the night staff came on. For the first time all day, they actually made an effort. They came to talk to me, see how I was and generally be of some help. There was a great comfort in their presence, not just to me but to all. The effects of the pills were still quite strong, so I was tiring fast and felt able to at least try to get some sleep. It had been of great relief in the past week or so that I was able to lose consciousness with some ease. Nevertheless, they gave me some more of those small yellow pills that had failed me so utterly, to hasten the process. Sleep came and in the morning they were gone.

Confused as time had been in the other hospital, in the Palace it went crazy. There simply was no concept of time there. We simply knew that it must be evening by the presence of those two caring souls that were our nightly sentinels. The absolute nothingness of that place merely exacerbated the sense of timelessness. All we knew was that we were there and it was beyond our control as to when we left, whether for good, or just a temporary respite for a few hours.

In the morning I managed to get out of the door for the first time. They told me that it was policy for them to keep people in for the first three days so that their condition could be observed. But there was no observation in here, only neglect. With the heavy door open for a change, the seer took me out with him. In view of their obvious lack of interest, and the fact that they never seemed to know who was there anyway, we just decided to out go for a while. He took me around the labyrinth that seemed to go on forever. Downstairs was the man and his eternal question. The seer told me he was always there, and that his name was John, although, as with every other story in the place, I had no idea of the validity of his statement.

Everywhere we went looked the same. Our path took us along the same chess board flooring, and above the pipes seemed to show us the way. Every so often, we came across old abandoned fire grates, a long defunct relic of its previous days. Doors were everywhere, and although many had signs on them, they made little sense to me. They merely added to the still growing fear of that place. My mind raced as to what the purpose of these hidden rooms was. All I knew was that like the small room at the entrance of the ward, I didn't want to enter any of them.

He was a kind man the seer. He said he'd been a police man and that he had visions of the future. He gloried in his belief that he had been of great help to his employers in predicting bombings and accidents. He's quite mad. I'm here, am I mad too? Thoughts coming back. They may have been disturbing, but at least it was a break from Rachel. She'd been very quiet in my mind, but the thought was always lurking. Maybe the excess of the drug had done me some good, but I was certain that as the effects wore off over time, she would return with a vengeance. Funny though the seer's stories were, and as genuinely believing of them as he was, at least we were away for a while, not only from the ward, but the wearing conversation of the old man there. The seer was easier to cope with.

Most importantly on our travels, he took me to the small shop where it was possible to at last buy cigarettes. It was staffed by a pair of what seemed like octogenarian ladies who did voluntary work through the auspices of the Royal Women's Voluntary Service. Their service was most invaluable to us all, but I did question their motives for being there. It was hard not to think they had been doing it for years because they felt it was their Christian duty to help those poor afflicted souls in this place that was supposed to help them. They were very kind if a little deaf and they had to stick by the rather quaint policy that only light brands of cigarettes could be sold so the health of the patients didn't suffer too much. It was a concession by the NHS, but an ironic one. Having made my purchase, we again headed off on our travels into the gloomy unknown.

By a circuitous route, we somehow arrived back at our starting point. No one seemed to notice either our leaving or our return. Nothing happened there except at tea time and meal times. We were just left there most of the time.

In the coming days it was rare that that door was open. There was little or nothing to break the monotony. I tried in vain to read to pass the time, but I was neither physically nor mentally able to undertake a task as simple as that; the *Chronicle of James I of Aragon* was now but a fleeting and distant memory, although in real time it was barely two months before. My parents came by sometimes but failed to let on their concern at the complete lack of care in the place. On their first visit I said something about it not really being full of my kind of people to which my father's response was that perhaps I needed to be with such people. This angered and scared me, but he, like me, was struggling to make sense of this place and was merely trying to find anything to say in the circumstances.

With boredom and this incarceration came tension. Arguments about things that were real or imagined were frequent. Occasionally blows were exchanged which was about the only thing that elicited a response from our guardians. These problems were far less common in the evening when at least someone was there who really cared; this correlation seemed to be lost on the rest of them. I lived in eternal fear; fear of my own demons which started to return the more the effects of the drugs wore off, and fear of the unpredictability of our joint circumstances. With that fear grew the desperation to get out but the feeling of utter impotence in being able to achieve that. I knew that being there was actually making things worse rather than better, but there was no indication of when or how I was going to get beyond that heavy metal door. It was a feeling that almost everyone seemed to share. The timelessness of the place exacerbated the problem.

However much I longed and craved to get out, in the back of mind was the thought that I had nothing to get out to. Locked up though I was, the suicidal thoughts were still there; Rachel was still there and unresolved; home would always be home; and I was virtually bankrupt. There was no way out except death and, as during the course of the summer, that would have to wait. But it was going to come, of that I was sure and determined.

Late one afternoon they called me into the office. I was left alone with a man who was in his mid to late twenties. He seemed tired but had a kindly face. I had a vague memory that he had been there that first afternoon, one of the questioners. He was better dressed than the others and was inevitably of more importance than those I saw on an everyday basis. He kept the meeting brief:

"I don't think you need to be here. You can go home today."

Relief overtook me and blotted out all else that he said. But with the elation there was the question of exactly what had been the purpose of me being there in the first place. They had done precisely nothing to help my condition, and the incarceration had actually made things worse. It appeared that little thought was given to what next, merely an outpatient's appointment in a couple of weeks. Yet in the moment, those thoughts were secondary. The arrangements were made for me to be picked and I set about getting ready. The others seemed very pleased that I could go home, the talkative old man, the guy with the psycho eyes whom I doubted would ever get out, the drag queen, the foreigner. And then there was the seer who told me he had had a vision and knew that I would go home that day.

The clanging of the iron door was both a relief and a sadness for me; I was going but they had to stay behind. John was again guarding the corridor as we left for freedom. But what sort of freedom? It was all the same. I had been there but a few days yet the experience had damaged me beyond even my own comprehension; just one day was one too many. There was the sense that I was now madder than when I had gone in there. Nothing had been done in the way of treatment and the future, apart from the pain I suffered everyday, was far from certain. But as we drove off down that bleak tree lined road to reality, I had a new determination. I was never going to allow myself to go back to hell in the Archbishop's Palace, and that meant that I had to get everything right the next time.

A Pillar of Impotence

Whatever the faithful may think of suicide, sin or not, nothing could be worse than that unholy place, with its Holy name. Especially not death.

Chapter 10

Reeds and Lilies

It was idyllic down by the water. The reeds masked my presence by land and water. A carpet of interlocking lilies set out before me across the still water, the bright yellow flowers still there, glistening in the late summer sun. The woods behind and the old war time pill-box extended the disguise from the path above. Ducks and swans passed from time to time, and snakes sunned themselves on the warm banks. Interruptions were rare there. Every now and then the tell tale clank of metal on metal distorted the peace, followed by the swish of the oars; these were the intruders who disturbed my private contemplations. This was my new refuge where I stayed for hours, unnoticed by those passing except in the boats. Here was as close as I could get to peace, but it was a peace surrounded by her echoing voice. Here I contemplated my individual turmoil; it was my place away from reality.

With my Kafkaesque nightmare physically over, at least for the moment, I was left with all from before but with the added problem of the reality of circumstances. Escape from the Palace was exquisite but it had its consequences to face. How could I hide what had happened when one look in the mirror told another story? How to admit that I had been to that place to those whom I would soon have to face, but who would have no conception of it? Almost immediately after my release from captivity, my mother told me that Rachel had been on the phone to find out what was going on. I had no recollection of anything, but somehow I must have got word to her that catastrophe was looming. My mother had volunteered the knowledge that I had been in two different hospitals and left it at that. But it was clear without even contacting her that she knew what had happened.

A more immediate problem was what to do about the invitation to see Becky. I knew I had to go just to get away but I was acutely aware that it would not be easy to have someone in my state to stay, but desperation was the better part of good sense. Having spoken to her, she still wanted me to come and arranged to come over from Sussex to pick me up. By the time she got there with another friend

A Pillar of Impotence

I was ready to run out the door as fast as I could just to get away. Knowing that they needed to know the truth, I was brutally honest with both. Neither seemed very surprised but both were well aware of the lead up to this point, and both knew Rachel and what had happened. There was a feeling of guilt that I had to put them through this, but I had to try to put it to one side. Out in the real world of the news, the Russian coup was still all over the papers and TV, but to me, it might as well have been going on another planet so far was I removed from reality; it was just something I stared at blankly on the screen.

My fears for their well-being proved to be right. My stay was marred by problems. The room in which I stayed had a photo of a smiling Rachel attached to the wall just above my head. That image gave a physical incarnation of what existed in my mind. With her above me, the sleeplessness returned with all its previous vigour, haunting the gradual hours of the night. While others slept, I was in torment. The waking hours were no easier to deal with either. For the second time since graduation I was gripped by an intense panic attack that made me seize up entirely. Unsure what was going on, and with me unable to communicate at all, Becky feared another overdose had taken place and it panicked her also. Although recovery was relatively swift, it was clear that we couldn't keep up the visit.

I knew I couldn't really stay after that but I couldn't face going back earlier than planned and was almost begging to stay. It was just a question of balancing needs. Desperate as I was, there was no choice. Ros went some way towards dampening the damage by arranging for me to go up to see her in London a few days later, but it did little to relieve the gloom within me as we drove inexorably back across the county border to the sea.

The time in Kent was slow to pass and excruciatingly painful. The few days before my next departure saw me wandering about aimlessly, shuffling down the road like some crippled wreck to my place of peace; always back to the water for some brief respite. Along with the insomnia the headaches also returned with the same intensity as before; the drugs now failed me in a second way. The stomach pump had been painful enough, but the effects of the little yellow pills had the ability to anaesthetise me from some of the excesses of the mental process. Yet that started to whither away on my return. I yearned to go to London to see Ros just to escape circumstances. The few days seemed to double in real time, but I got there in the end.

I had a post-relationship relationship with her. We remained quite trusting friends and she had the crucial advantage over most people in that she had insight into such problems. When we were together, her foibles had mystified me, but now that I was there myself, I began to appreciate both them, and what support she now had to offer. Above all though, I was away from some of the pain except what I took with me inside my mind. Her family were also very understanding and very kindly arranged for me to meet a private psychologist for whom her mother worked. For the first time I came across what always seemed to be a curious trait of such people: he insisted that I had to phone up myself to confirm that I wanted to come rather than for someone else to do it. Since I was developing an increasing fear of telephones this proved very hard for me to do. Amid a great deal of stress, I was able to make the call into the unknown, then, late in the afternoon, set off to see him.

We talked for a while, and for the first time, someone who was a professional talked to me with some sort of compassion and care. I wondered if this might be a sign of the private sector but said nothing. We talked of the state that things were now in, at that minute. We talked of suicide and what it meant. We talked of the future and what that might hold. He gave little reaction to much of what I had to say, but at least he listened; that was rare in my experience. He suggested a couple of places local to me that might be able to help me and then we parted. I tried them both subsequently and neither could help me, but at least someone seemed to be with me rather than against me; that was partially gratifying.

The one thing that disturbed me about both my meeting with the professional, and my time with Ros, was the habit they seemed to have of underestimating what was going on. The words "it's only depression" that I heard frequently exacerbated my feelings. Although probably meant as a reassurance, it seemed to me to be a betrayal. Like those others with whom I had had contact, they seemed to share the view that this was a temporary condition that would clear up after pills and a bit of talking. I seemed to be the only one that recognised the complexity of the situation. Even at the first meeting with the bearded man, I had been relieved and disturbed by his summing up of the situation. However, this did not take away from how thankful I was of their efforts to help. My time with Ros was all too short, but under the circumstances, I found a little peace there. But then, as always, I had to go back.

Ros and Becky were quite trusted friends who knew me well and I was able to be entirely honest with them about what had happened. But I had to face the rest of the world at some stage. Above all, I had to speak to Rachel. We talked briefly on the phone and arranged to meet up. By that stage she was living with a friend in London which also brought the difficulty of what to say to her if she wanted to see me; one look would give away so much. I both relished and dreaded the prospect of seeing Rachel again. We had not met since our parting at Cambridge station a couple of months before and clearly the world had changed since that point in time. I was in turmoil by the time I got off the train to wait for her. I had to do all I could to stave off another of the panic attacks I suffered now with some frequency. Then she arrived and some sort of order was restored to my shaking mind and body.

She displayed no reaction to my appearance and just talked quietly about not much as we moved off in line with my slowed motion delaying our progress. My squinting eyes hid behind shades as I tried in vain to mask the pain in my eyes and head. Neither of us really knew what to do as we walked to Covent Garden for lunch, but I sensed that she, like me, was trying to map out what would unfold in the ensuing play. She took me to a small but cosy vegetarian restaurant in the market. It would not have been my choice, another of our many differences that seemed so important to her, but I went in with good grace.

"Talk," was the single word that she uttered as we sat down.

In a way as calm, dispassionate and non-guilt inferring as I could manage, I allowed the events that had happened to come out. It was very important to me that I moved as far from giving her a sense of blame as was possible, but it was hard. How could I get away from the reality that it was her actions that had driven me to the course of action that I had taken? How do I avoid telling her that when I still loved her? At the same time, it was hard to imagine exactly what she was feeling. Yet she listened with her usual compassion. She spoke sensibly, and explained that the only reason that she hadn't come to see me as she had promised was that she had left her address book behind and had no number. I had no real reason to doubt what she was saying but was struck by the irony that something that simple had been the thing that had finally tipped me over into the abyss.

Despite the compassion, the veil that had existed for most of the last year had come back. The shutters behind which she had hidden for so long were firmly back in place. The apparent progress we had made back in Cambridge had been blown away in the magnitude of subsequent events. It was rarely to come down again in my presence in subsequent years except for the occasional slip when things were going wrong in her life. She still cared greatly, but seemed determined never to let me back in on a meaningful level. Perhaps that was a natural response in the young.

Our afternoon together continued in much the same vein until we went to meet her housemate. Rachel had asked me if it was alright to tell her, but even though I knew her and she had been there that afternoon in the coastal wine bar the year before, I couldn't face telling her. We spent the rest of the time together just as friends meeting for the first time in a while and talked the crass bullshit of such occasions. How much she knew she never let on, nor did she comment on my physical condition; another who simply did not know what to do or say so she simply hid behind the small talk.

I sat on the train back utterly despondent yet content that I'd finally managed to catch up with her. Confusion reigned, mixed with the realisation that I was headed back to my own private oblivion. I didn't know at all what I was supposed to feel or how to deal with what was a deeply traumatic experience for me if not for her. I headed back to the nothingness that had become my life. I took with me the memories of the day and her voice, that quiet echoing voice.

Life settled back into its pattern, long, painful and disturbed days followed by even more painful nights, then the wake up call. Each day was the same. I moved around very slowly between my cell, my place and occasional visits to town for no particular reason. My only reason for anything was just to get away for a few hours. I tried to mask myself from the world as much as I could, wandering aimlessly in a semi comatosed state, eyes shaded from view. I must have presented a curious sight to those out and about. I passed the mums collecting their children from the nearby school each day but saw them not. What they must have thought of this strange fellow I have no idea and it never really crossed my mind. I was anonymous here and that was how it had to be. Each day seemed to take a week to pass. I had to fight each minute just to get through. I often felt like screaming and destroying things but that would only draw attention to me and I couldn't deal with that. I just turned it all in on myself, and that only continued the cycle.

I had an Out-patient's appointment with the doctor shortly after I'd seen Rachel but it produced little of note to help me. He was as evasive in his responses as they'd all seemed to be but he had got me out of the Palace so at least he had done something. Still confused about what was wrong with me, I asked him what he thought about the idea of it being depression but all he said was that it would be more evident if it were clinical depression. I wondered how much more evident it could be than that which had happened but left it there; I was still in the dark and in doubt. I'd not had any more pills since I'd left the Palace, so he put me on some different ones which he assured me were not dangerous and would help me sleep. They, like the previous ones failed. That pretty much set the pattern of our meetings over the next couple of months.

"How are you?"
"Worse." Always the same, just the pills changed from time to time. Other than that there was no treatment, just another appointment in two weeks.

At the end of the month I turned twenty two. My sister and brother in law came down for the event, and they took me out for dinner at a fine Chinese Restaurant which had been a favourite of mine for many years. I was entirely distracted throughout, thinking only of death and that I'd never make twenty three if I could possibly help it. In the middle of dinner which had been dreadful for me so far, I had a devastating mood swing that took me into the absolute depths. There was no reason for it, it just happened. These unexplained swings, a movement between different depths of hell, became a constant feature of my as yet unexplained condition. I had no control at all, and with that, the fear grew ever deeper. I had no reason to celebrate that day but had to go along with it. People's good intentions often made things worse. All I wanted to do was die.

The following day I had to face the world for real, and these were people who were unaware that I was ill. I had agreed to sing at a wedding in Sussex on the last day of August. The horns of a dilemma were before me: be exposed to the world and escape for a day or be stuck in pain at home; I chose the former horn. Exhausted as I was from days of not sleeping, the drive down there was precarious. I was one of the last to get there and found everyone waiting for my arrival. I could see the shock and questioning on their faces as I got out of the car. Each face emitted the expression that said "what the fuck has happened to you?" They didn't need to speak and few did, the few questions getting the mumbled response that I had been ill. That was all I could muster. Singing was much harder than it had ever been so distracted was I. Staying focused on music was almost impossible, so much was going on in my head, but somehow I got through without running out. The reception was worse. No one really knew what to say but they all wanted to know. I fought off the feeling of panic several times, and then turned for home having promised to see everyone in a few weeks.

The journey back was even more arduous than going and I was forced to stop. I sat alone in a graveyard in a small country town alone with my thoughts. Different ones kept rushing at me. What to do. What to say. What did they all think? Above all else was that I had to go back now. Rachel spoke and the tears came, hidden from prying eyes by my ever present shades. In despair I undertook the last part of my journey. Round one with the world was over, and I knew that it brought more questions than answers.

Life at home returned to its norm of nothing. In addition to the mental anguish the physical side of things continued to worsen. It was like having a permanent hangover. My head pounded for all the waking hours. My eyes hid behind the almost closed lids desperately trying to blot out the day light; rain or shine it was the same, shades hid me from the world and the world from me. All day

I was shattered and the sleepless night only made it worse. At one point they decided to put me on powerful pain killers but they didn't touch it so I gave up. My thinking moved on to a physical explanation of the pain. The exhaustion gave some credence to the idea that it could ME, the disease of the time and one far more acceptable than the apparent truth. There was also a desperate desire for it to be some terminal illness, not as they were later to tell me that it typical of a depressive illness, but because it seemed better to die with honour than to die of suicide. Anyway the head pain was just too great to be psychological so we looked into neurology; if nothing else, it gave me hope for a while.

All the while I sought as much as I could to travel about. This was of course limited by my precarious financial situation but as long as I could get some help with petrol I could still get around. Mid September took me back to Sussex for a large reunion with old school friends. I'd had a life saving offer from one such friend and his family to come down whenever I wanted for a few days just to get away. Over the years Trapper was to prove my redemption many times, a fact for which I will forever be grateful. Again it was exposure to the public as a whole but it was better than being stuck at home. I drove down with my usual trepidation to find that the news of my illness had spread rapidly. However, there was an overwhelming sense of support from all and sundry although they were all bemused by what was going on. I spent an exhausting but pleasant day with Rachel and others. All seemed concerned but powerless. Rachel was fine but still guarded and little was said between us. My return was the same gloomy affair as normal but at least I had had a break.

Within days however, my Doctor heard of my visit and instantly stopped me driving. And that was the final springing of the trap; there was no escape now. With my isolation now utterly complete, things got even worse. My withdrawal from the outside world continued. I spent my time huddled and shaking in my sacred place, tormented by the eternal mental music and her voice. Suicidal thoughts ran riot tempered only by the hope that might lie with the neurologist. I sometimes wandered aimlessly into town, shambling along engrossed in my anguish. Rachel's birthday at the end of month almost drove me over the edge again. I found myself fighting and crying all day and not knowing why. I had no desire to live so why fight the urges? Then at night I sat in front of a faceless TV barely comprehending what it was all about. My nights were no longer filled with the revelry of the pub that had been my norm for so long, I had neither the money nor the stomach to drink any more; drinking just made me feel even worse.

Slowly, as the summer slipped into autumn, the carpet of lilies and the blanket of the reeds diminished denuding my cover. It was almost imperceivable as the foliage died off, first the yellow flowers closed up and drifted off to the shallow depths, then the shrinking started. No longer did I have the noise of inept oarsman to interrupt me. That part I liked but losing the camouflage added to my sadness. My feeling of exposure hung heavy on me as it got colder.

September turned to October and I fought on for no purpose. Towards the end of the month I managed to scrape together enough money for a train ticket to Cambridge. What should have been a respite turned into a disaster. When I got to the college I found that they all knew the truth. The American from Ohio had met one of my friends in the States and had talked. It was common knowledge and only suspicion accompanied that truth. Having left them in the evening I stood for a while at the old house in West Road. It was locked and hostile. I suddenly felt away from home. What had always been home was no longer. I couldn't deal with them knowing the truth and I'd lost my one true refuge. None of them really knew what to say to me and nothing was ever said openly. But if it was like that with those who had lived with me for some time, what would it be like to meet new people and hide such a secret? It proved to be one trip away from which I had no solace only harm.

I did, however, locate a brief modicum of solace on Sundays. This was not Sunday solace that an ever decreasing number of the population, Rachel included, found in the church, but in my great passion for American Football. I'd been acutely aware that when I left Cambridge there would be no more football, but, shortly after I left the Palace, I'd stumbled across a junior team that played locally. I'd set out to coach and help out as much as I could but I was limited. My attempt to put on the pads and helmet again had proved to be utter folly, but just being around there and at games helped just a little. For a brief few hours each week I was almost able to blot things out of my mind and immerse myself in something I really loved. But there were many hours in the day, and there were many days in the week. Time was infinite, football was not, but I welcomed all the diversions I could get.

As time rolled by there was no sign of any breakthrough. People I passed in the street frequently told me that I looked better but this annoyed me. They were just saying it to be polite. My meetings with the shrink came and went in the same vein as before; the same things were said and the pills were changed but none of them made any discernible difference. They seemed to all think that I was a bit depressed and I would snap out of it after taking some pills. No other effort was made and it seemed plainly obvious to me that if that was what it was I should have responded by now. I knew they were wrong but no one seemed to listen to me. In my meetings with the shrink no mention was made of trying something new, they just didn't seem to give a shit. On and on it went, nothing ever changed especially not my desire to get out of there, and only by dying could I achieve that cherished goal.

By November my hiding place was almost bare. At that stage it had turned wet and muddy but it didn't stop my daily journeys there. The conditions kept all but the hardy and the dog walkers away. That was a good thing. I hated people intruding in to the only real space that was mine. My routine carried on as it got darker. I sat alone with my mental exertions as my only company, a shattered wreck of what had once been a creature of such promise. There was no help for me, and there was no hope. Loneliness was all I felt, and once again I was nearing the end. It will soon be over. The thought echoed in harmony with her voice. Soon Mark, soon.

Chapter 11

Movement

It was sunny that late November morning. Alone I huddled on the back step smoking a cigarette, rocking rhythmically back and forth and trembling. It was always hard to know whether it was the cold or the illness that made me shake so much but it always seemed to be there. It was cold but the rays of sunshine warmed the garden as they were wont to do as the morning progressed and the sun moved round from east to west. It was a more pleasant experience than it had been of late there but I still struggled to get the filter tip to my lips. My mind was ablaze with activity but that was normal. Today was looking to turn out just like any other, a fight from start to finish. Nothing was planned and nothing out of the ordinary was expected. Then the phone rang and disturbed my focus. Panic set in. Although I often had calls from friends wanting to know how I was but I had started to develop a fear of phones and it was unusual for calls to come through in the morning. Unsure what to do I staggered slowly into the house. It kept ringing despite my slow speed of movement, each ring and each step adding to my anxiety. I picked up the hand set and was confronted with an unfamiliar woman's voice on the other end.

"Can I speak to Mark please?" Who's this? What does she want? Why has she disturbed me? The thoughts came in an instant.
"It's me," was all I could muster in response.
"My name's Suzanne and I'm from the Day Hospital."
What's that? Where is it? Why are you calling me?
"I've been asked to call you as we thought you might like to come along."

Getting this call totally out of the blue threw me. At last it seemed that someone was doing something, but what was it? I felt some relief that there was at last some movement, but with that there was a great deal of trepidation at having to face others in an unfamiliar environment.

Much of the rest of the conversation passed me by, but at the end she gave me an appointment to at least come and view the place later in the week and then hung up. It left me with very mixed emotions and more confusion. More thoughts to add to and conflict with those already there. I feared my own state but I feared the unknown even more. Could I handle it? What could they do to help me? Could they help me? More questions but answers would have to wait; if there were any answers.

A few days later, I was driven to another destination previously unknown to me. There was a modern annexe attached to a hospital of similar ilk and age to the Palace, my old college and my old school. Everywhere I went I seemed to end up in Victorian buildings. To the right of and above the annexe were large ponds at which a few hardy souls could be seen fishing even this close to winter. I'd never seen what drew people to fishing, but whatever it was, it must have been good on a cold day like that. A sign outside ushered us into the annexe area. A large and airy waiting area opened up before us with doors going off seemingly in all directions. It was reminiscent of all the doors at the Palace but far less forbidding. We approached the reception desk with a draw down grill above it and announced our presence and appointment time. The receptionist acknowledged us and asked us to take a seat.

Two rows of about half a dozen seats faced each other in a regimented symmetry with a small, low table covered in neat piles of magazines. We sat down in an atmosphere of uneasy silence. Two people sat opposite us, and in that peculiarly southern style we failed to converse and avoided eye contact. That was, however, entirely normal for me now; from that very first day I never could look into anyone's eyes.

The woman was older and beautifully dressed, but with a great sadness in her face. He was young, younger than me, with swept back dark hair. He was sitting but it was clear that he would be very tall when he stood up. He looked painfully thin and had his head deeply buried in a book as he seemed to be intent on blocking out the world from his thoughts. Whatever was going on inside his head appeared to have completely cut him off from all that was around. A mother and son awaiting the call just as we were. It would be the two sons who were about to enter another unknown portal. I knew not his story, nor he mine, but it was clear that the next part of this torrid journey, we would undertake it together for a while at least. It transpired that his name was John and it would take us about three months before we realised that we lived all of fifty yards apart.

A double door creaked open at the end of the seating area and a woman emerged to invite us both in; she was Suzanne. Inside was a large area with many seats, a pool table and various other bits of equipment. Seated there also was another woman. She was much younger than the Suzanne, about my age with blonde hair and an unusual eye that unnerved me. She introduced herself as Vicky, and, between the two of them they explained what was done there and why they wanted us to be there. Vicky said that she was an Occupational Therapist a profession of which I had never heard, and tried to explain the difference between what a nurse did and an OT; it didn't make sense to me at all, but at that stage it didn't seem to matter. It seemed that they offered a series of what they called groups that were supposed to help people in our position. I held out little hope of there being any shift but at least it was worth a go and someone seemed to be doing something. I was told that Vicky would be my key worker for the time I was there and she arranged an appointment for me to see her later in the week at which a programme would be worked out to fit my needs. They seemed to be very keen on fulfilling my needs but as it worked out, it was only them who decided on the input of what my needs were. After what seemed like an age we emerged out into the same area to see the mothers talking; I guess they had had nothing better to do but it made me nervous. We then headed off respectively to our own abodes blissfully unaware of our habitual proximity.

Amid a sense of great nervousness I went along for the first time to their social afternoon. I said that I'd try it for a short while but was of course hampered by a lack of transport, so I was there for the duration. There were all kinds of weird and wonderful people there: the drag queen who served the tea; the loud; the confident; the quiet; the timid. It was a melting pot of differing forms of humanity brought together by that extraordinarily diverse concept that people like to call mental illness. It was a fearful collection but that very binding that linked us all gave a sense of welcoming. Unlike the Palace I felt some sort of ease for and affinity with these people. We were all in it together whatever our personal circumstances. I was struck by the number of them that I had seen wandering around my home town on my travels; it dispelled the idea that I was totally alone. The staff were equally diverse, some friendly and approachable, others aloof and distant. The latter exuded a feeling of you are them and we are the professionals so keep your distance. Sadly Vicky proved to be one of the latter.

My fledgling relationship with Vicky was fatally compromised the first time we met one to one. She seemed to have a problem with Cambridge and informed me that "just because you've been to Cambridge it doesn't mean you know about mental illness, I know about it, I've studied it." The impact of the statement which came unexpectedly was immediate and devastating. Here was a women who it turned out was only a few months older than me and like me, straight out of university, imposing on me her own insecurities of where I had come from. Fury reigned in my head. I couldn't give a fuck what she had studied, I was living it. That was what mattered to me. I'd never felt I knew what was going on and had come there for help not to be told foolish things like that. We would meet every week for the next two years or so but the damage had already been done; no relationship of that kind had a hope of recovering from that. Worse still I was to be stuck with her. There was no facility to change unless a worker of the opposite sex was required. She seemed to make great play of the fact that she was a woman, intent on knowing whether I minded that. I didn't give damn as long as they were prepared to help me. That was never to happen with her.

The problems with Vicky aside, something was better than nothing. Going over there three or four times a week got me out and away from the place I most detested. Much of the alleged therapy was a complete waste of time, art was a question of paint a picture and you'll feel better, but I had too much time on my hands so it filled in for me. Above all it was contact with people who had some sort of idea where I was coming from but in a much less oppressive way than at the Palace. Most of the people I met were very friendly and willing to share their experiences. Others were very guarded so it was better to stick to the maxim of the man I had met who told me never to ask what was wrong with people. That was a kind of unwritten rule here too, but it was one that didn't bother me. The day and night, however, were very long and the groups short. Each time I finished I dreaded heading back. Then there were the weekends. Nothing to do and nothing to alleviate the pain and boredom. Football on Sundays consumed some time but never enough.

At around the same time as my unexpected call up to treatment, I got what I had been dreading for the last three months or so, the call up from the DHSS. A lifetime, and indeed, almost a death time had passed since I'd first stumbled into their office to be told I had a week to find a real job or just take anything. Every two weeks I had had to make my way into their soul destroying establishment to tell the untrained operative in the glass cage that I hadn't done any work in the previous two weeks and then sign on the dotted line; only then did I receive my pittance. They knew that I was ill as I'd had to miss an appointment to sign on whilst in the Palace but had said nothing. I'd feared the day when they were to check on what I had done to "seek work" to justify my enormous expense to the tax payer. Throughout that summer and autumn I had vaguely and vainly tried to get a job purely to keep them and everyone else happy. Nobody seemed to take any notice of the fact that there were neither jobs to be had nor that I was clearly too ill to work. Then came the brown envelope through the door, summoning me on pain losing what little they gave me, to appear on the prescribed date.

Anxiety and panic began to grip me as I waited there. I had a few meagre bits of paper and letters of rejection, hoping desperately that they would be enough to keep them happy for a while. I just managed to prevent myself having another panic attack as I was called in and surveyed suspiciously by a woman I'd never met before. She asked some questions and looked at the paperwork provided. It proved to be enough for the time being, but another time would come and that was another three months away. My trauma now temporarily averted, I mused on exactly why I was required to do all this and be at their mercy when it was so obvious to all who saw me that I was ill. Yet no one offered to help or even look into it. I merely stumbled along in troubled ignorance having yet more pressure put on me by some faceless bureaucrat who was just following the instructions to get people off benefits and so make the figures look better.

Through all of this there was little or no change in my condition. Pills came and went along with the doctors. The man who had got me out of the Palace went and was replaced by a woman from Germany. She was young and friendly but seemed to have no more idea of how to move on than any of the others. My head was still pounding, my eyes still hooded. Sleep seemed practically non existent. My mood was always very low and merely fluctuated between certain parameters. It could just go for no reason or shift in relation to outside forces. Every time it took a turn for the worse they wanted to know what had caused it; only rarely could I pinpoint anything specific as a cause. My frustration and feeling of hopelessness was relentless. Death and suicide pervaded my thoughts, and Rachel and the eternal music invaded my mind and senses. Yet as we moved into December and Christmas loomed large and dreadfully, there was a little glimmer of hope. There was an appointment with the neurologist set up if only because we went private.

It was a freezing Saturday morning when we set off to another place that was unknown to me. In order to maximize his profits, he had decided to see me at 8 a.m. which was the last thing I needed having been awake well beyond 4 a.m. The house and its location were testament to the earning power of those who work in the private sector. It did not seem that his wealth extended to heating the place; it was almost as cold inside as it was outside. He took me into a large and equally cold room and proceeded to question and prod me for about twenty minutes. Then came his answer.

"I can find nothing wrong with you neurologically." That much I could deal with but it was his next comment that overwhelmed me.
"You're just a bit depressed. Why don't you go to Italy for a couple of weeks and you'll feel better?"

I was stunned. My mind went into overdrive. Who the fuck is this cunt? £75 to be insulted. I didn't come here to be insulted. What fucking cretin would suggest that? What fucking planet is he from? Had he ever been trained to deal with real people? My thoughts turned to my previous attempt to get away to clear my head; France had been great in its own little way but had done nothing to alleviate the illness. Now here I was over a year later and much further down the track of madness and this was the best that medicine could offer. The irony would have been funny were it not for the fact that it was so obscene. As we drove away into another day of hell through the freezing mist of the valley, I mentally resolved that it was time to finish it once and for all. This time I was determined not to fuck it but wasn't sure how to do it. That would come to me in time; I had another weekend get through and that was more pressing and immediate. And with that, the headaches that I'd sought to alleviate went on.

The impact of this man's sermon lasted for many days. The turmoil peaked as badly as it had ever been before. It was a two-fold disaster: I couldn't deal with the patronising way in which he had made his announcement, it was yet another reinforcement of my belief that nobody cared. It was as if they had done their job by saving my life against my wishes and were now going to let me rot in my own cerebral filth. Secondly, and more importantly, it took away my desperate hope for death with dignity. The rage and desire to end things soon began to take me over again.

A few nights later I went out on one of my nocturnal forays. Completely locked into that mode I broke down outside in the street. Through an endless stream of cigarettes I felt a sudden and unexpected block on my thinking. Something in me made me realise that at that time, I could no longer go through with it. The desire was there but the ability was not. It seemed that for a while at least, those around me would get their wish and I would live. I hated that block and began to despise myself more. I had lived in a constant state of suicide since June, now I couldn't go through with it again. I had failed and had no chance now of rectifying that failure. There was now no way out. Death had been my only hope for so long and now I couldn't reach it by any means. I made my way back in the house and collapse on the bed utterly distraught. Yet again though, sleep refused to come.

Chapter 12

'Tis the Season to be Jolly

There is something about Christmas; whatever the circumstances, people always seem to celebrate it. The banal comments that we make to each other concerning our health switch to comments about Christmas. What are you doing for Christmas? It's a time to be with your family. Have a Happy Christmas and New Year. Our very demeanour changes at that time of year. It is as if it is some beacon in the middle of winter that most of us feel we have to enjoy; whatever problems there are in our lives, we try to put them aside for that brief holiday. So it was that even in the depths of recession, troubles were ignored and the celebrations started with the putting up of decorations in the street, and people girded up their meagre resources to buy presents, cards, food and drink. That sent a terrible signal to my mind. What the fuck did I have to celebrate?

The run up to Christmas had actually started quite well for me. I managed to get a trip up to Cambridge early in the month and finally witnessed my old team beat Oxford. Despite my weakened state, that was something to celebrate. I paid the price though the next day. I was really too ill to be there, often passing out in the day and unable to get any sleep at night. I had many friends in town that weekend which was great but I couldn't keep up with them. I took them on the King's Street Run, but a pub crawl when one is ill and not drinking creates all sorts of mental turmoil. It was the first time since I'd left that I'd been in a party atmosphere and not joined in; I was completely lost. Not long after my return I was thrown into similar circumstances with equally confused results. The Football team in Kent had a post season party for the players and coaches and helpers. It was heading into the unknown again; none of them knew about the illness. Questions were of course asked about why I wasn't joining in with the drinking. More excuses had to be made; the cover up never seemed to end. I had planned, and dreaded, to stay up there but with a great deal of relief I managed to get a lift back and get away. It set the tone for all future gatherings. Invites in the future became a source of fear and trepidation rather than of joy, and each would bring more lies to be told. The secret had to be kept.

Things slipped rapidly downhill after that. The season became more and more isolating. Despite the problems with Vicky and the limitation of what they had to offer, the Day Service was a refuge of sorts. That, of course, would be shut. The prospect of seeing no one at all loomed large in my thinking. All the signs of coming festivity weighed heavily. People seemed determined to enjoy themselves without thought of the consequences but that put more pressure on me. It was as if it was expected that all troubles be forgotten and fun was to be had. Yet I could not forget at all. I had no control over my thinking or anything else that was invading my mind. So soon after stumbling across the unexpected suicide block, this sense of expectation was too much to bear. Not only was that a problem, but it was the anticipation of the Christmas post mortem that was to follow. No one could have done with Christmas, they had to keep banging on about it for weeks afterwards. Then there was the expectation of going to church on Christmas Eve. I had no desire whatever to go anywhere near a church for the foreseeable future, yet I knew the enmity that that action would elicit in certain quarters. Everywhere was pressure to do what I hated, and that was to live and enjoy it. I was alone but not alone. All I wanted was to sleep right through the whole thing, just blot out the fact that it was happening. But my mind would not let me do that; it simply sought to punish me.

As I went out late on Christmas Eve I took another route; church was nowhere to be seen in my thinking. On a cold but windless night I slipped quietly down the hill towards the sea. I had determined long before that this would be another of my nocturnal wanders but this time it was secret in another way. There were great signs of celebration from the pub at the bottom of the hill but no one marked the route to notice my passing. What is there to celebrate? What is there to celebrate? Over and over in my mind, temporarily blotting out her voice. I moved at my usual slow pace along the road that led directly to the sea. No one appeared. The voice started again as I meandered along. The tide was low when I got there and I climbed slowly down the precipitous stone steps onto the slipway the preceded to the shingle. It was calm and clear, just the quiet sound of the waves broke the silence. The sounds of celebration were far back in the distance. To so many others, peace was reigning at that spot on that particular Christmas night. There was no one there to witness the calm or, more importantly, me.

A Pillar of Impotence

My mind was afire. Thoughts fighting with the voice. The voice would override it and then lose its power. Waves of thoughts swept me up into an ecstasy of despair. Then the voice came back. It echoed as it came, sometimes loud, sometimes soft matching the creeping whisper of the waves some fifty yards beyond my spot. With the pain came the tears, and with the tears came the music. Each section of the torment vied for precedence like maestros trying to outplay each other. There was a desperate desire to die. I just wanted it to stop. Yet I was drawn to the place to be alone, and being alone meant this maelstrom. The mental block that had come up so recently rose again. Like a thirsty man deceived by the mirage, I could see and feel what I wanted but could not get there. Desire was there but the capacity to do it was taken away. The thoughts were almost taunting me.

I don't know how long I stood there in this trance like state, but I was eventually aroused by the knowledge that I needed to get back before everyone else. People interfering and intruding again. My mind carried on its battle as I headed back at the same slow and methodical pace. There was no let up back at the house, just another sleepless night to follow. That night set the tone for so many subsequent Christmases. It became the time of year when I was at my worst, and there was nothing I could do to stop it.

The New Year dawned a week later. It had absolutely no impact on me or my state of mind. It was to be the year in which we would all become European. No one seemed to want to be European but, as with so many things in this country, little heed was paid to what the people actually wanted. It would also be the year in which the Tory government would be re-elected to the shock of so many. In the east war rumbled on. It was still early days in the Balkans and we had yet to use the term Ethnic Cleansing in every day life. The town of Srebrenica was still unheard of in the west. It had been less than a year since Desert Storm but George Bush's proclamation of a new post Cold War order was already looking like a fallacy. That fallacy would be borne out as the decade progressed. Of more pressing consideration were the dire economic circumstances in which we found ourselves. For a short while I was safe from that but it would not be long until the inevitable brown envelope came through the letter box and added to the pressure again.

Life returned to what seemed to pass for the norm after the New Year. It was a minute to minute, hour to hour existence. I returned to the Day Service on several days of the week but made no progress at all. The treatment on offer continued to fail but talking to those around helped me to make some sort of sense out of my afflictions. I talked but above all I listened. People rarely if ever asked direct questions on what was wrong, rather that they talked of symptoms.

"Do you hear voices?" That question again. Back in the summer when the bearded man had asked me the same thing, I hadn't understood what he meant. The words were simple but its meaning and my ability to conceptualise it was lacking. Now people started to explain to me what it was like. It slowly dawned on me that Rachel's voice was some sort of variation of this but did not seem exactly the same. They talked of unknown voices tormenting and ordering them to do things. In other cases people seemed to suffer from a barrage of criticism. It all sounded very frightening to me. What I heard was specific and recognisable but not really threatening or critical. It was more of a haunting voice, reminding me of my self. Where the cross over came was that it was incessant and out of my control. Sometimes she was quiet although still always lurking somewhere in my head. What was disturbing to me was that it was a constant reminder of the things that had come to pass and there was no respite from that. The past was replayed constantly with either that voice, or, occasionally, through very vivid flashbacks. Yet my fear of the Palace, reinforced by the words of the others kept me silent. By that stage it was what I lived and expected and I could see no benefit to be gained from talking about it.

The great benefit of the place was the sense of camaraderie amongst us. Whatever our afflictions, diverse as they were, we were all suffering and apparently powerless against illnesses that few of us understood. In our own limited ways we supported each other. An aspect that seemed to run through most people's experiences was the feelings that they were being treated poorly. Many had been through years of this System epitomised by the dark disaster that was the Palace. People's fear of the place was palpable. Like me, many were reluctant to talk of what was really going on out of fear. We feared the power of those with whom we worked. There was little or no trust of the professionals. For so many of us they were, in effect, the enemy. Many, like Vicky, were young and inexperienced and seemed to have little understanding of how we felt. I knew straight away that it would be impossible for them to empathise with people who had mental illness but few even seemed to try. There were exceptions; the co-ordinator was a wise and kindly man who cared a great deal. And then there was Jack.

I knew as soon as I met him that Jack was different. He ran fitness groups at the centre and I met him very early on. He took time to get to know people. He never pushed people beyond what they could safely, or more importantly, comfortably do. Above all else Jack took time out to listen. He made us all calmer and then allowed us to relax without some hidden agenda. I never really felt better from exercising although many others did. What really set him apart though was the fact that he'd lived mental illness. He was one of us, and he was trusted for it.

The New Year was barely a month old when the expected brown envelope dropped through the letter box. I was summoned again to explain why I was apparently of no use to society other than to take money off it. It felt as if I was just a drain on society and that I had to justify my existence. Fear came at me in another form. What shall I do? Will they take away what little they give me? Why are they hounding me? More thoughts adding to the usual confusion. It was a few days before I was due to be summoned to explain myself that I was having one of my regular meetings at the GP's surgery. I mentioned my fears to him and got a very unexpected response.

"That's okay, I can sign you off sick."
"Can you?"

He took out a small note pad, filled in various formalities and put the word "depression" in the space for diagnosis. It was that simple, for the next three months I would be safe.

A great feeling of relief flooded over me. But it was tainted relief. Why didn't they tell me this before? Over and over the thought came. With it came anger. It was not an anger aimed at him, just anger at yet another example of the total fuck up that seemed to characterise the actions of those who were supposed to help me. I had spent six months feeling pressure that was absolutely unnecessary. All it would have taken was one small piece of paper. What little faith I had left that anyone actually wanted to help me was shattered, it just seemed like another betrayal from the medical profession. I didn't express the anger, I merely turned it in on myself again.

A few days later I wandered gingerly into the depressing offices of the DHSS with my small yet significant piece of paper in my hand. A woman called me through and motioned for me to sit down.

"Before we start you'd better read this."
I handed over the piece of paper. She took it and scanned it for a few brief moments.
"Have you any idea how long this is going to last?" was her opening remark. I was taken aback by this. I was incredulous. What a stupid question I thought to myself. Another example of their complete lack of care for anything other than to get me off there books.
"I've no idea but I've been ill for well over a year."

She took out some paperwork and began to fill things in. She took the form and just told me that was all she needed. I had no idea at that time how significant this was. No one had told me that if one was sick for more than six months one was entitled to more money in the form of a disability premium on top of the normal benefit. In fact, no one had told me anything that was of any use. I had been sick all the time that I had been signing on, the appropriate six months, but would not be paid that money until the paper work had been processed. It wasn't even clear that I would get all the money to which I was entitled. I might even have to wait another six months. They did eventually pay me for that first six months but it did nothing to relieve the memory of having to look for work when I was too ill to do anything, nor the hassle and wasted money I spent having to go in once a fortnight to sign on. It merely added to the web of distrust and betrayal in which I was now entwined. I was still being let down on all sides. The first battle with the DHSS was over; there would be many more, and they would become much more complex and drawn out.

February turned to March and still there was no real progress. Slowly the effects of the drugs still there since August began to abate. The only real change was that I was more awake and with it than I had been. This was mistakenly seen as a sign of progress in the illness. But reality was still there even if that only seemed apparent to me. Nothing had changed in my mental state and it was becoming increasingly clear that not much was working. My doubts about their opinions, such as they told me grew. My weeks were now filled up for a few hours most days, but it was never enough. The hardest time was still as the day wore on. Mornings were bad but afternoons showed a slight improvement. For a few hours I was a bit more aware of what was going on. Yet as those afternoons wore on, the deterioration started as I headed toward those terrible nights. I was seeing Vicky once a week but my distrust of her was strengthening. The shrink from Germany saw me once every couple of weeks as did my GP. None of them told me very much; I was giving but not receiving. I had but one hope: the coming of Easter brought another choir tour. It was all I had had to look forward to since leaving the Palace in August. Much as I relished that prospect, I knew it would be all too short. Yet a week was a long time in my existence where that time seemed to be forever standing still.

Then there was a shift. An appointment was made for me to see a consultant for the first time. So far the two that I had seen had been more junior, and although the first of them had got me out of the Palace, their efforts had been ineffective. It seemed to me that this had to be a step forward if only because a consultant would have more experience so I was relatively optimistic.

I went to the appointment accompanied by Vicky and the German. It took me back to where I'd met the bearded man on that first day. The meeting proved most disconcerting. He barely spoke to me. He listened to Vicky, then he listened to his junior. At no point did he refer to me about anything that was significant. He gave the impression had he had no interest in anything I had to say. Then came his conclusion. I was to return to my original pills but in much higher doses. This time they would be bigger and pink. He wanted me to undertake a lengthy course of Psychotherapy. I was to learn later that this was called Cognitive Behavioural Therapy, but the term meant nothing to me. There did seem to be some sense in the first two parts of his deliberations. Then came the final part. Vicky was going to concentrate on helping me back to work. There it was again, the "your depressed because you don't have a job" syndrome.

It was another total misunderstanding of what was going on. Although his intentions may have been good, the mistake was made again. This from a man in power, a man who had no interest in what I had to say. I was, of course, bowed by my own ignorance.

On the surface, it appeared that things would be moving forward. A new and more vigorous approach was being tried, but deep within me, I knew there would be more problems ahead. I had a woman whom I didn't trust controlling my treatment and by extension my life. She was young and inexperienced, and more importantly, had already compromised the working relationship. Then there was the man with the real power, and he wouldn't even talk to me. That aside though, maybe just may be, it would have an effect.

Prague was now just a couple of weeks away. Those days took forever to pass. As the countdown started, I began the new medication regime and the Psychotherapy. It was not, however, to be conducted by a psychotherapist. The psychiatrist from Germany was to do it herself. I never ascertained whether she was fully qualified to do it. There was some debate at the beginning whether it would be recorded or not; they decided against it. Another psychiatrist was to supervise it, but they never told me exactly what that meant. It was all very vague and it felt as if I was stumbling around in the dark. I still foolishly believed that they might know what they were doing.

Chapter 13

No Longer Alone

When singing as a young child there had only been one reason to exist; being the best there was the be all and end all of our world. Nothing else mattered but that. Mistakes were not expected to happen; that was unprofessional. The pressure was immense but that was what we were used to even though most of us had been only eight or nine when we had started. The pressure came not only from those who sought to profit from us but also from us. In a way we were conditioned to be like that. That conditioning was backed up by extreme, if rare, violence. Even that seemed normal to us; we knew no different. We just lived with it and hoped each day that that would not be one on which it would be unleashed. When it came to singing, that legacy still held sway with me. I just put the pressure on myself now, but that was enough.

I had sung at a few concerts since getting ill but going in tour in my state was a much more daunting prospect. It would be the most sustained period of having to focus on music since our trip to Barcelona the previous Easter. Although I was very ill then too, it was before I'd broken down completely. Then I had struggled to get through and finish Cambridge in the medium term. Barcelona had been a wonderful if pained distraction. I had borne my secret better in those days. Now I had to face many people for an extended period of time looking obviously ill. Few of them knew that I'd been ill. Even fewer knew the truth. Then there were the new people that I'd yet to meet. Above all, I was no longer able to be what they always expected of me on these trips. I was always in the forefront of these trips, partying as much as anyone. That wouldn't happen this time. Despite these fears, I had been desperate for this time to come for many months. It was the one thing I had had to look forward to in what was an increasingly bleak present and even bleaker future.

The trip followed its usual format of gathering to rehearse for a couple of days before making the journey. My struggles started there, although those around me were largely unaware of that fact. I was still having problems with reading and that applied to music as much as literature. More mistakes than usual occurred, and, as I would have expected, that was very difficult for me to deal with. There was frustration, but above anger at myself. I couldn't operate at the level I had always expected. I'd always felt that part of the key was being reliable and helpful to those with less experience. That had always been part of the way we operated. Now I was letting them down, and my own ego, but it was my feeling, and I alone had to bear it. I had to rely on instinct and memory just to get by.

Yet it was the evenings that would be more difficult to bear. These trips had always been characterised by the enjoyment we all derived from them. We worked hard when we were performing and rehearsing and then we played hard. It was as much a social event as a musical one. In this respect it differed greatly from the music I'd done in Cambridge the second time around. The lack of enjoyment of what I was doing was one of the main reasons for giving it up. Now, after a long day of work, I sat quietly and detached in the pub. All around me, my colleagues passed the night away in our usual manner. It was as if I was in a dream world where I could see what was happening but I couldn't connect to it. People tried and failed to get through. The pretence of normality was too hard to keep up. The despair began to creep in; I had looked forward to this for so long but it seemed to be all going wrong before we even left the country. Exhaustion and headaches clouded around me. For the first time since I'd been touring there was no enjoyment to be derived but at least I was away from home.

For the first time when flying I experienced some anxiety. This had more to do with the rickety nature of the Russian-built airliner on which we flew than any sudden development of fear but it was palpable nonetheless. The hotel was unlike any I'd been in before. It consisted of a series of apartment blocks each divided into reasonable sized flats holding up to four people. They put me in an apartment separate from most of the others so that I'd be able get away to a quiet area if I wanted to with an old and trusted friend. He knew some, but not all, of what had transpired. The arrangement suited me well but for the drawback of being on the fourth floor. It would prove indicative of how badly things had hit me physically that I could barely get up and down those stairs. Once up I had to rest, and my corresponding descent had to be made very early before the times needed to allow me to recover. More than once my room mate had to go up for me for things I had forgotten because I was too exhausted to make the climb. That proved a shock to me and added to the sense of fear and helplessness.

Prague as it turned to spring proved a staggeringly beautiful place be. The climate was just on the turn on our visit, snow the week before, then warm sunshine by the end of the week. Despite the obvious poverty of so many of the people, the place was vibrant and happy. People smiled wherever we went and there was a great sense of being welcome. It was also absurdly cheap in comparison to what we were used to, yet far too expensive for the legions of students that we met along the way. The food was rich and sumptuous and we dined for next to nothing. It was a Westerner's paradise with all comers taking advantage of each other. To us it was a bargain, to them it was hard currency; it suited all of us.

Its beauty and friendliness aside, Prague did little to help my strained mind. The omens had not been good whilst still in England and my fears and frustrations became stronger as each concert and day passed. The quality of my own performance was severely lacking. No one said anything but they didn't have to. I was my own judge and a harsh one at that. With each mistake came more self hate and anger. The schedule was far too much for me to cope with and further exhaustion followed. My concentration was virtually gone and at one point I had to leave in mid concert. I sat alone outside this particularly grand church in the dust and wept behind my ever present shades. The music strained on behind me in my aloneness but did nothing to distract from that within. My mind raced away with thoughts of regret, and above all, failure. Part of me wanted to just go back but that was an admission of defeat. It would have been very hard to organise and I was in no fit state to travel alone. And besides, I had nothing to go back to. As the concert drew to its close, I knew I had to get back to some sense of normality; there was still a great need to keep thing secret. The mask came back and the excuses were made as they emerged from the gloom that accompanies so many churches before we headed back for the next part of the agenda.

Yet it was not the business side of the trip that was most difficult. The times when we were off duty were always the hardest. Night time had always been party time on these trips, a time to wind down after the day's work. It took us to the bars and Beer Halls of the city having eaten in some splendour. My place had always been at the front, now I just reverted to the background. Each night we went out and it was the same. People were always trying to check that I was okay as I quietly sipped soft drinks and thought and brooded. Only rarely did a glimpse of my old self emerge, and then it was very brief. It was as if I were a bit part in the performance that was played out around me. I had just become part of the scenery that they didn't quite know what to do with. As the week progressed the frustration began to turn further to anger. I'm a burden. They wouldn't notice if I slipped quietly out. They don't need me here. Go back. My thoughts ran away from and in on themselves. Much as part of me wanted to just run, that was impossible. I'd almost completely lost my sense of direction and fear of getting lost in a strange and dangerous city was far greater than the apparent joys of the alternative. Likewise, I knew that it was far better to be with people, even those to whom I felt I meant nothing, than being alone. There, the thoughts were in danger of taking over completely. Then, when we all headed back to the apartments and the inevitable extension of the frivolity, my lethargic and shuffling turn of pace would slow them all down. And that was another imposition on them in my mind. With each passing day my mood got steadily worse.

On Easter Sunday a new dilemma was thrust upon me. We sang a morning service at a church and were looking forward to the rest of the day off. Those who smoked did so out of desperation outside with echoes of *This Joyful Eastertide* still ringing mentally. People mulled around considering where to go for lunch or which bar to attend for the afternoon as we waited to make sure all was well. Then came the news that I always dreaded on these occasions. The congregation and various local musicians were staging an Easter concert that night and wanted us to take part. Such extra performances were rare on these tours but not unheard of. Four year before we had accidently stumbled across a service in Seville Cathedral that was to draw some 5000 people and be broadcast live throughout Spain. But that was when I was well and could take such things on easily. Now was another story. As always, it would rely on those with great experience, and of course that meant me. Exhausted already, I was now confronted by a two hour rehearsal and new music to learn.

In the event, that rehearsal stretched me to breaking point. I had to just resort to instinct and simple guess work. We had to learn the whole of a Haydn Mass in an hour as well as various other things. Fortunately the predictability of Haydn did come to my rescue, and somehow I made it through the afternoon. I was amazed by the sheer talent and musicality of the local Czechs; they were quite brilliant and so natural. The event itself went exceptionally well, much to the surprise of many of us taking part. Even the Mass was almost flawless. Then it was over. I'd survived. I even had a feeling of satisfaction and accomplishment that I'd not felt for many many months. The feeling only survived about an hour of the evening. Then it was back to reality as the black beer of another Beer Hall was vehemently consumed by all those around me. Joy never lasted long for me.

People always tended to divide up into small groups when not singing unless it was late at night. It allowed us to discover a wide variety of hostelries and to share information for use along the way. It was, however, our custom to always go out together on the last night to eat in whatever establishment best suited our purposes. This was affectionately known as the Last Supper. It was always a memorable event for all, but one that held great symbolism for me, both good and bad. Prague would be no different to normal. We had discovered a small restaurant near the hotel whilst out for someone's birthday earlier in the week. It was a curious place, its entrance guarded by a heavy wooden door with a small opening that was opened after loud knocking. We'd eaten a tremendous meal there for about £5 served by an eccentric Serbian who made us laugh a great deal, and, referring to the quiet, unobtrusive and old background music had informed us that Abba was "great music to fuck to". The restaurant was not due to be open on the last night of our visit, but we'd persuaded them to open just for us for the Last Supper. It was only just big enough for all of us but would suit our needs perfectly. By that stage I'd had about as much as I could take. Not only had the trip been a personal disaster, I now faced the prospect of going back to my usual existence. Confronted with both of these problems I decided to give in and join the rest. I knew that physically it would make me feel instantly worse, mentally I could at least banish the pain for a few hours. It was time to drink again. Although none of us realised it as we went in, it would prove to be a fateful night, one that none of us would forget for a long time, if at all.

It was a typically celebratory evening after the success of what had been my fourteenth such tour with one group or another. With the strength of that which I imbibed my old public self re-emerged much to everyone's delight and above all expectation. There had been moments even on this most harrowing of trips where it had appeared. Yet then it had been fleeting, false and too hard to maintain for long. Now, for tonight at least, I was back in the land of the living. My head pounded even more than ever, but the mental anguish became veiled and muffled with each glass as it slowly drifted away from my conscious. By the time meal was coming to a close and the speeches, presents and thank yous were approaching, I was splendidly drunk. The atmosphere was cheerful and boisterous as they went ahead with much interruption from the throng. I found myself talking to someone I hardly knew. It was a chance and unlikely remark that changed the night for me. I have no idea why I said it but it just came out. There were so many there who knew me well yet knew nothing of the truth of the last few months.

"I took a massive drugs overdose last August." To an almost complete stranger I'd come out with the truth out of the blue. I'd kept it hidden from most of those around me. I stunned myself with my own voice. Yet it didn't stun her.

"I think I need to talk to you" was her instant response. There was no shock and no emotional response, just a one line answer. I'd had no inkling of it that week yet I had stumbled upon another traumatised soul. We said little more of any significance as the party carried on. We didn't need to say more, we just had to wait. The rest were oblivious to what had just happened as they had been to so much that Easter. We were all also oblivious to the drama and catastrophe that was to unfold in the early hours of the following morning.

Fuelled by cheap wine and beer, we returned to the hotel intent on carrying on the party. It didn't have a bar but held a number of well stocked fridges in the lobby. These were plundered with relish on our arrival. Yet we didn't follow the crowd. Almost unnoticed, I slipped off with my new found confidante towards the other apartment area armed with two bottles of champagne. The long climb up to the fourth floor seemed so much easier now. My exhaustion was blotted out by the occasion and the alcohol. I didn't care about the physical pain any more such was the strength and volume of the anaesthetic administered in the pleasant surroundings of an obscure Czech restaurant.

To the accompaniment of champagne our respective stories came pouring out along with a great deal of emotion. Those stories differed in many respects yet we shared so much in terms of the impact that these events had had on our respective lives. She was utterly alone never having told a soul of what had happened to her. I was not quite so alone; some knew some of my story, others knew more. There were people nearby who knew much but none really connected to it. That is what transpired that night, an absolute connection, empathy and understanding of two vulnerable and traumatised people. I learned much that evening about myself and the nature of emotion and life. I had a sense of power over what had so far rendered me powerless. Talking really did help but only to one who understood. I listened, I understood, and I helped ease pain; she did the same. Although I talked of Rachel I was never troubled by her voice or any galloping thoughts. She understood my pain, and I hers. A great calm descended over me. It was peace, a peace I'd only ever envisioned in death. For the first time in nearly two years I was at peace and I didn't fear for the morning. We didn't care about what was going on elsewhere, we were simply content where we were. We talked on late into that night, then came an untroubled and easy sleep.

I woke early the following morning. My head felt like I'd just been hit by a train. Yet that peace that was so alien to me was still there. I didn't care about the physical, just the mental. She slept on for some time as I just lay there enjoying the moment. I had always hated waking early as my mind invariably came alive and started to torment me as soon as it happened. Today it was different. I had two hangovers, one good, one bad. The good easily outweighed the bad. My mind wandered in the silence of the early spring morning. There were only good thoughts. Going home to England and all that that entailed was far from my conscious. She woke sometime after me and we chatted quietly as we both got to grips with that morning after feeling.

I don't know what time it was but there was unexpected knock on the door. Time aside, it was still early for the last morning when we didn't have rush to the airport. I walked down the passage way wondering who it might be. To my semi surprise it was Becky. We exchanged such pleasantries as we could, then she unveiled the reason for her visit.

"There's been a terrible accident, David has fallen out of a window." The impact was instantaneous. I knew that he, like the rest of us, was staying on the fourth floor, and that the chances of surviving such a fall were remote to say the least. She knew little else of what had happened apart from the fact that he'd been rushed to hospital. There was a meeting arranged for not long after so that the facts, such as they were known, could be passed on to the rest of us. With that she departed.

We dressed hurriedly in a stunned silence. When she had headed back to her own apartment, I set about packing up and preparing for what I knew would be a harrowing scene. Any residual effects of the night before were banished, but I was struck by how unusually calm I was. Troubled though the times were, the peace and calm I'd achieved remained. I was shocked but it was as if everyone had been catapulted into my world. Life and death had become my world. I felt a sudden usefulness descend upon me. I was on familiar ground.

I found a group of shell-shocked people when I went to the meeting. Details were scant but it seemed that he was in going into surgery and that he was unlikely survive. People wandered around in a daze not knowing what to do or say. It was compounded by the realisation that within a few hours we would be leaving the country and would be reliant on the phone. Steve and Neil were to stay behind but the rest of us were to go; few of us wanted that but there was little choice. We gave what comfort we could to each other but there was an air of futility to it. I spoke to many in as calm a way as I could but there was no telling what impact it had.

A few hours later we boarded a bus to the airport. The journey was fairly quiet, just a few people trying to take their minds off things. I'm sure more that a few people silently prayed for his survival. It was hardest on those who had shared an apartment with him. They had been woken by Czech police asking amongst other things if any of them had pushed him. Fortunately, there was very little delay at the airport and we made it back to London without incident. The other thing that most of us dreaded was also by-passed, there was no interference from Her Majesty's Customs. Unsure of what communications were like from Prague, I phoned Steve's parents from the airport to put them in the picture; they already knew. Then it was back to Sussex to wait anxiously by the phone for news.

I stayed down with Trapper for a few days afterwards. Fresh supplies of the pink pills were sent through the post. We met up and waited what seemed like an eternity for news. The comforting still went on as the hours ticked away, the trauma still very much in evidence. Then it came. By some miracle David had survived. There would be many months of pain ahead, but he was going to live. He would eventually mend and begin his life again. I was still there when Neil returned. He'd felt it more than any us; he was solemn, quiet and aged.

In those few short days in Sussex I mused greatly on the vagaries of life and fate. Here was me desperately yearning for a death that never came, and this young man who cheated it by chance when it unexpectedly arrived on his doorstep. It was very hard for me to deal with personally. He had not, as we feared, been a victim of excess, in fact, he hadn't drunk at all. As far as could be ascertained, he had tried to open the window when sleep walking and fallen out. Fate could be cruel in so many ways.

Prague impacted in so many different ways on so many different people; I was merely one of those many. Yet its impact on me was unexpected. Faced with crisis I had coped surprisingly well. More importantly though, I had taken the first step forward. It was only a tiny step but it was palpable. I was no longer alone. I had made a connection that was lacking with those I knew at the hospital. Not only that, I had done something to help someone else. There was at least one person out there who could see where I was coming from. The hard part now was finding someone who not only understood, but had the ability and power to help me through. None of those I'd met before had that, and I now faced going back to my painful existence alone again, and back in their power.

Chapter 14

Itinerant Madness

Prague was but fleeting experience, but one that was to herald a new period of frantic travel. I constantly ran from myself over the next few months but I never could succeed. The extraordinary events of the trip and having to deal with them faded quickly in many respects, all that remained was that David was stuck in hospital for many months and was apparently getting better. That in itself was comforting but I could not seem to get myself any better. My mood was still uncontrollable and deeply low. The pills did a little to alleviate the sleep problems but no more than that. Rachel was abroad and I heard only intermittently from her. That worried me but there was little I could do about it. She was, however, ever present in my mind. She and everything else were my constant and painful companions on my travels. When I did hear from her there was always a paradoxical mix of joy and fear. Letters would arrive and lay unopened for days, so fearful was I of the potential contents.

The other constant in my life was therapy, whatever that was supposed to be all about. After a very short space of time my doubts about it had been confirmed. All I seemed to be doing was giving out vast reams of information for little or nothing in return. It was as if the German was doing research for a book and I was her primary source. I had no real idea where it was going or what I was supposed to feel about it. I certainly never felt enlightened or any better for it. All we did was drag up things that were already clear to me. Having insight seemed to be a dangerous business when it came to psychotherapy. But then again I had always had that insight even as a young child. I dreaded the weekly sessions and rapidly lost any faith I had in it.

She did, however, do me one great service. After many months of relative immobility, she relented that I could drive again. There was the proviso that I kept my journeys to short distances. Although this was a limitation in the wider scheme of my itinerant life, it did allow me a modicum of local independence. I was no longer indebted to anyone to travel to and from the hospital and I had the ability to get away more. Local towns were now within my grasp without a price to pay. It was a small but significant shift for me, a little triumph.

Spring moved into summer and memories of the Palace and its bars came back with the heat. Things deteriorated rapidly in June. I crossed the suicide line and was only brought back from the edge by the efforts of Sophie and Becky at much cost to themselves. There were repercussions this time as people from the past actually made contact with my GP to warn of my condition. I was furious but powerless at that.

That fury was rapidly intensified when the German announced that "you're not ill, you just have a lot of problems." Where she got that idea from I had no idea but that seemed to be the line she wanted to take for better or worse. It didn't help me very much, simply alienating me further and instilling even greater distrust. Vicky was also widening the gap between us in our weekly meetings. The end of anything meaningful happened when she told me that "you do have to want to get better." Her line was that I could only do it myself but I was completely lost. I couldn't see what I had to get better for and I knew that the views of the experts were failing me. I now severely doubted their ability and their diagnosis. I could accept that I had very low mood and was essentially depressed but I felt it was more complex than that. It did not explain the violent mood swings or Rachel's voice. The fear of every day living and those around me still abounded. My head pounded constantly and there was no explanation. Above all, if I had depression, why on earth did I have no response to the treatment? I didn't know it at the time, but the shrinks were having similar thoughts but heading down a new path that was so far from the reality that I lived that it was scary. But that was to be in the future; I wasn't yet ready to realise about the hidden agenda that accompanies most cases of psychiatric treatment.

Treatment of that variety was still the unmentionable in my life. Rarely did I have to face my old world in Cambridge but when I did it brought other fears. Like the paradox of Rachel's letters, so I was drawn to Cambridge knowing the pain it would cause. Suicide Sunday that year was one of those enigmatic experiences for me. There was an intense sense of loneliness as I mingled through the usual drunken crowd. People all seemed pleased to see me but lost as to what to say. Awkwardness hung in the air around me as I tried to celebrate what had traditionally become the great day of the party year. The Pimm's flowed but not down my throat. To many the sight of drunk people when one is teetotal can be amusing; to me it was just painful. There was a desperate desire to just run, but I had nowhere to run. The hopes I had for the day that I could wile away a few hours away from my personal torments evaporated quickly. Then there was the inevitable lying. The truth, such as it was known, was a casualty of the day. I was with those I had been closest to for three years but there was no joy, just melancholy. Too many memories of too much pain. My forlorn looking house seemed to peer at me from around the corner. The gardens were beautiful but awful. Thoughts of past times flooded my conscious mind bringing waves of sadness; Cambridge was no longer mine as it had been for so long in my life. I was but an exile now with no real hope of getting home. We punted late in the afternoon to my old haunts in Grantchester, but there was no respite. Tiredness, only tiredness; that was all I felt. Why did you come? You don't belong here any more. You deserve what you suffer. The thoughts never shut down, even as I tried to sleep at night. I was mentally and physically exhausted but no sleep would come to me. There was much to regret about that weekend.

There was a certain inevitability, given my and own condition and the company I kept, that my journey would take me back to the Palace sooner or later. It happened that summer. Matt was a young man who I'd met very early on at the Day Service. In his ever present leather jacket he'd been one of those who struggled and toiled with art. He was the first to ever mention the word that people in the real world feared most, schizophrenia. I was initially struck by his youth although it was to transpire that he was, in fact, two years older than me. To this day he retains his youthful looks despite the traumas of his life. He was quite open in his ways without obvious fear of stigma. But there was little fear of stigma when we were with our own people. He was a deeply disturbed man who fought a terrible, valiant, and largely unsuccessful war against his voices and the physical and tactile hallucinations that plagued him sometimes. Yet he was always there for others and I learned a great deal from him particularly about voices. What I experienced was rather different to his own experience, but he did help get things into some sort of perspective. What I didn't know about Matt, and was to learn this much later, was that he enjoyed immense support from his family. His mother worked tirelessly not only for him, but for many others as well. I would meet her very soon but the connection was not made until later. As I saw him, he was a rather isolated figure who struggled to live in flat somewhere near the hospital. How wrong I was.

When Matt was taken into the Palace I was faced with a terrible dilemma. He was my friend, and as such, I had no desire to leave him to face that place alone. On the other hand, my fear of it was immense. After much deliberation, I decided to put away, or at least try to suppress that fear and go back. Then, of course, I realised that I absolutely no idea where the Palace was. All I knew was that it was somewhere near Canterbury. Armed with instructions from Vicky, and fighting my own lack of direction, I set off on an alarmingly warm afternoon, alarmingly similar to the conditions I had faced that previous summer. At least though, I went this time with the knowledge that I could walk out of that door when I wanted to do so. That was a great comfort as I headed towards the place I feared more than any other I'd ever been to.

Spotting the dilapidated houses along the road was the first sign that I was on the right track, but with that, my fear became more palpable. I swung into the tree lined avenue with its paradoxical beauty and drove slowly up to the old Victorian building. Heart pounding and my thoughts going I was just about able to hold it together by just repeating silently to myself "I can get out whenever I want." Over and over it went as I approached the once glorious entrance hall. Some way to my left was the entrance that I had used that previous summer; it just made me shudder. I didn't know where Matt would be so I asked at the desk, then it was back into the labyrinth and its accompanying gloom. The stench of despair and decay was still all pervading; nothing had changed. After some time and much confusion I came to the door with the specified name. It was locked. Pressing the door bell, a woman in her thirties opened the heavy metal portal and allowed me in. Nothing stirred in there in that oppressive heat. I could see bodies in bed there was nothing to tell that these poor people were alive. The stench was appalling. I asked for Matt.

"Never heard of him" came the answer in a thick Scottish accent. "How long has he been in?"

"Not long" I said, "he came in last week."

"This is a long term ward. Try back at reception."

It was a horrible thing to hear. It was hell on earth there for a few days; for a life time, it didn't bear thinking about. She scuttled back to her office and I left as fast as I could. Somehow, through the labyrinth, I found my way back to my private hell; he was where I had been kept. Sweat poured off me as I rang that bell. It was hard to tell if it was the fear or the heat that drove this automatic bodily response, perhaps they were just vying with one another. At least I can get out again. The thought came back. Hang onto that. They opened the shutter, then the heavy door swung open and creaked as it went.

"I've come to see Matt."

"He should be around somewhere" came the disinterested response. He led me into that familiar area, the place of tea. "Try the TV room." With that, he wandered back to his office. That was also familiar.

I meandered through getting quizzical looks from the people I passed. There he was, alone and silent. The TV was off and Matt just sat there staring into space.

"Hello Matt." There was a time delay before any response, he continued to stare off into the distance. Then he head shot round and he came out this strange trance.

"Sorry about that" he said, "I was just in a room full of people and they were all shouting at me at once." The room was empty and it was only now that he realised that. This was often the norm for Matt. The voices ruled his world. He was shut down from the world as I was but in a far less lucid way. I pondered on which was worse.

It was hard to stay calm in there, there were so many terrifying memories, but I had to for his sake. I stayed for over an hour then said my goodbyes and left. As I left the building I could feel the tension dissipate, as if sweated out through my pores. But that relief was tempered by the guilt that I was leaving Matt there. There would only be an escape for him when they chose it. Fortunately, he seemed to cope rather better than I did; he was used to it. That was my first return there. I knew as I drove away that other trips were only a matter of time.

The visit to the Palace was one of the more traumatic of my jaunts around the country, the one that I didn't really want but was forced to take. But like the difficulties of Prague, I had survived. It troubled me to leave Matt there but at least it wasn't me this time. I wondered who would come to see me were I to be put back in there, but at least I had some belief that I would not be left there like last time. That would always stay though. It was back to the norm of my existence from then on.

At around the same time I made a discovery of great significance; there was more help out there. Miriam had spent some time trying to research what was available other than the ineptitude that I had suffered up until then. We found that there was a group that met once a week under the Aegis of the charity MIND. There was still trepidation as I prepared to go, but I went in the knowledge that many people that I already knew were there regular basis. It was a Wednesday evening group that was there for all those who suffered. What I found was very different from what I was used to; there was support but this time it was unconditional. There were no hidden agendas attached to it. We were free there without being under the constant gaze of those we didn't trust. That was something of step forward and it would become a regular haunt for me. Another place to get away for a little while and be with those who really understood. They also cared.

As summer drew on there was another change. My father took up a job in Scotland in August of that year which meant that he was really only there every second weekend or so. The real difference though was there was less shouting going on and fewer arguments and a sort of fake peace descended on the house. Of course the constant complaining, judgement, and bitter barbs continued just without its usual target there.

I still had the remnants of the cricket season to see me through the day. The little things that could distract me for a short while were very important. Although many hate and misunderstand the concept of a game that went on for five days, to me, it was a great distraction. I struggled to focus and forgot much of what I saw but it was something between my journeys that I could do. With the coming of autumn, life was revived by the arrival of the NFL season but I could see much less of that than the Test matches, and nothing live. Winter would then bring the Five Nations. They were small things that occupied only a few hours each but they were the pegs on which I hung the mantle of my madness. Travelling after all was only finite; I still had to return each time. And it always came with me.

The drift from summer to autumn brought relief from the heat, the daylight, and its accompanying glare. It also completed the disillusionment with the treatment that I was receiving. It had been a year of broken promises there. So much they had to offer was made off limits to me. They had mentioned Art Therapy at the start but dismissed it without even talking to me about it. Then there was the possibility of taking the advice of a psychologist. Vicky went to see him without me and that too was dismissed without my knowledge. It just seemed to go on and on. At no point was I even remotely involved in working on my own care, they simply dictated and presented their results as a choice. In reality, all their choices were loaded with no alternatives offered; I took it or would be dumped out of any support at all. By that autumn I had no faith at all in Vicky yet I could do nothing about it. She was still in control. The therapy had yielded nothing tangible. It seemed glaringly obvious that it had failed, the diagnosis was wrong, and I was going nowhere fast. They really didn't seem to give a shit and were totally oblivious to the pain I was enduring. The one exception was my GP. He was deeply concerned and seemed to genuinely care. Yet all his suggestions were ignored.

Nothing changed through the autumn or the winter. Christmas was the same disaster it had been the year before with me repeating the same ritual of the beach. New Year followed and the nightmare continued. The only real difference was that I was one more birthday down the line with nothing to celebrate. I could see no change anywhere, or even, what there would be for me in reality even if there was a change. I had my people and friends in the hospital, but nothing was changing for them either. It was not just me who was being failed by them, it was all of us. We merely had each other to cling to and exchange horror stories. Then there were the fears that we shared too. The Palace still loomed as a prison in our minds. Death and suicidal thoughts were everyday occurrences; the two were like brothers. Each of us who had those feelings also knew the price of failure was being locked up again. Yet we only saw each other for short periods of time as the norm. When the Service was shut, most of us went back to our isolation. Between my travels, both short and long, I was alone. Alone and without hope. Thoughts of the release that death would bring were my solitary companions.

Chapter 15

Chance Divergence

In the ramblings of my disturbed mind I often mused on the idea of chance and fate. Little things had brought to where I was now, and it was those little things that, had they been slightly different, may have taken me down another path. Chance had taken me to Rachel and all the consequences that that had brought me. I'd gone from a life where, to an extent, I'd been in control of what was going on. Now that was gone and I was at the mercy of my thoughts and voices. Life was just random now and in the power of others. I neither trusted nor believed in those others. They had also failed me. But I could see no alternative to it. In the early part of 1993 I started to cast my mind around towards finding another route but I had no idea where to look for that alternative. What I didn't know was that the vagaries of chance were about to strike me again, but this time in a better and more positive way than before. Fate would bring about that change that I craved but could not see. New people and new connections which would bear fruit in a limited way were still hidden over my horizon, but they drew closer as winter died away and the warmth of spring came.

It was quite the norm at the Day Service for people to come and go. Those who went rarely were much better than when they'd come in, and left for a variety of reasons. Some couldn't handle it and left quickly. Others just left because they got pissed off with the way that they were treated. Others still were discharged, often against their will. More often than not though, those who came stayed for a long time. All of this was testament to the futility of what was on offer. What our perception of what the place was about was radically different to that of those who ran it. To them it was a highly structured and specialised unit that was designed to rehabilitate those who were sent there. To us it was a place to go to fill our time and to be less isolated than we normally were for a few hours a day. Few of us had any faith in the group system that seemed to operate on the notion that if the patients could operate in every day life the same way as an average person could, then the job was done and we could move on. In practice, this essentially meant that if we could get up in the morning, wash, dress, eat, and get out the door, we were well. Of course, that didn't bear any relation to where any of us really wanted to be. The one real exception to that was going to Jack's fitness. He just had a special ability to work with us and a great affinity for our fears, pain, and lives. But Jack had lived himself in our world, and that made all the difference. Jack's was always too early in the morning for me, but I regularly went along if only for his company and understanding.

I was at Jack's one morning painfully going through his circuits and waiting for the coffee break when I became aware of a newcomer. He was strikingly young and looked a little confused. He also looked rather tired and very ill. When we got to the end and we all headed for the coffee and the cigarette packets, he came up to me to talk.

"What's wrong with you then?"

He's broken the cardinal rule. You can't ask that straight off. Thoughts came rapidly and confused me, but I was struck by how wonderfully uninhibited he was. Maybe it was because of his youth. Almost automatically I responded even though I was taken aback and didn't really want to say anything.

"They say I have depression." It was a guarded answer because by that stage I had no faith in that diagnosis and was convinced that they were wrong. Then we just got talking. What emerged was both startling and frightening. He was only seventeen, had been incarcerated in the Palace for the last three months and was only allowed out on the condition that he attended the Day Service. I was left so traumatised by my short stay there that I shuddered at the thought of what this man had experienced. That length of time there, at any age, was too much for me to even think about. At seventeen, it was unbelievable. How on earth had he survived? That was a thought that went over and over in my mind as we parted at the end of the session and he got his lift home.

It was chance meeting but one that would prove highly significant for me. Over the coming months James would prove to be a great friend who would provide me with another refuge that was just a short walk away, and someone to talk things over with at length.

More significant though, he would be the first person who would get me back out into the realms of what people called reality. I feared that reality as much as he did but together we started to go back to the pubs and public places that I had shunned for so long, but had been such a strong part of my previous life. Our paths had crossed almost by accident, but the next part of the journey would no longer be undertaken alone.

The good was quickly followed by more bad news. I started to have problems with my vision that spring. I'd been plagued by myopia since my early teens with my eye sight changing so rapidly I normally had to replace my glasses every six months or so. The rapid decline had been slowed a great deal when I started to wear lenses at sixteen, partly to do with vanity, but mainly to allow me to play sport at a more competent level; it was very hard to play rugby when I couldn't see the ball. The downside of wearing them was the maintenance. They were expensive, and, like almost everyone who wears them, I did cut corners. Then there was the painful moment when the build up of the protein on the surface of the lenses made them unwearable. One day they felt fine, the next I couldn't bear them. That had happened on that very first day of my madness. The solution was simple, just a process, but that took time. I thought that was what had happened that spring morning in 1993. I hadn't yet noticed that my vision was not right.

Thinking that that was what the problem was, I took them down for the prescribed enzyme treatment and waited for the next few days for them to call saying they were ready. I'd never seen as well with my glasses as with my lenses and thought nothing of it that my vision was more blurred than before. When I got them back, I put them in as normal. To my surprise there was still the same irritation as before and my vision wasn't right. The immediate thought was that they were wearing out and I needed to go back for an appointment to get a new pair. At the appointment there appeared to be nothing wrong with them. He merely suggested that perhaps the irritation and blurring had something to do with the medication. That seemed logical, maybe even obvious.

The next time I was at the Day Service I casually asked one of the staff if that medication could have an effect on my eye sight.

"It can't be that, your optician must have made a mistake. Try making another appointment" came the response.

That struck me as odd but not wholly unexpected given the response I usually got to my queries. I'd known my optician since I was about twelve or thirteen. He'd always been honest with me and helpful. I found it far harder to doubt what he said than what came from the people at the hospital. Nonetheless, I went back and made another appointment. Same result.

The pain became so great that I more or less gave up wearing them. This of course laid me open not only to intense sunlight, but more disturbingly to the world. My shades had always been my mask from both. I couldn't cope with people looking into my eyes and always averted my gaze from them. I was also having problems seeing to drive. The net effect as the weeks went by was a dramatic lowering of my mood. The car was a life giver to me; it represented the only freedom I had to get away. Now I feared that I would, once again, lose what little I had. Yet I was still getting the same response from those who were supposed to help me: it couldn't possibly be the pills.

About three months after the first symptom, I made a final visit to the optician. As I suffered the pain he inspected both the eyes and the lenses, and he noticed that there were in fact, signs of something on the surface of them.

"There's a film on the lens and I've never seen anything like it before. Whatever it is, it has to be caused by the medication."

That was enough for me. I knew I had to get off the pills. But it also brought serious implications for the remnants of my relationship with them. They had lied to me one more time. Now I had to persuade them that I had to come off the pink pills and see what would happen next. It was yet another nail in the proverbial coffin.

Reluctantly, they admitted that it could after all be the pills, and that perhaps I should come off them. The German decided that she could put me on a derivative of the drug that would help me with my sleep, but it was important to come off them over a period of a few weeks. That was a good plan but it was the start of another excruciating battle. It was a battle I'd not thought about but it was one that made my life even harder than it had been. It would take a few years to find out what was happening, but over the next few months I suffered awful withdrawal symptoms. Life became like one giant bout of flu. I couldn't eat without feeling sick. I never was sick but the even the thought of food made me nauseous. My weight began to plummet but once again there was no explanation. All they saw was that I seemed to not be taking the opportunities given to me at the hospital. To them I was taking up space that could be used by others. I didn't know it but they were formulating a plan that would make things even worse, but that would not become apparent until later in the summer. Things were shifting but I was being kept in the dark. That had not changed.

Pills and sight aside, other things began to happen as winter became a memory. At Easter my long awaited return abroad occurred. The memories of the trip to Prague, both good and bad, were still very vivid. But as with the year before, the annual choir trip was the one thing I felt I had to look forward to through the dark months. We were all in two minds as to what to do but it was felt that we had to go again if only to prove that we could survive the trauma. Cadiz was to be our base for the week as we travelled around Southern Spain for the third time in five years. I had my usual demons to face, but being slightly less tired than I had been in Prague, I decided to join in more than I had and try to bring back the old me even if it was fake. That, of course, meant drinking again, and there was a terrible physical price to pay for that. It was a price I was prepared to take as I switched into what I would always call "my choir trip mode." It proved doable for a short period and the trip was a great success marred only by the chronic sunburn I suffered at the end. There were slight glimmers of joy in Spain, even when not drinking. My mood sank somewhat as we flew back; another year to wait. That year would turn into three before we were to go again.

Around the time of my return, I discovered, via one of the other patients, a small, and above all quiet social club where I went occasionally. The loud was only manageable on tour. For the first time in nearly two years, I started to go out in the evenings. It was friendly place with few questions being asked. It was also very cheap. That was important as money was still very tight. I didn't go very often and never drank much. Even a small amount to drink still had a profound effect on my physical well being, but the mental effects made it a price worth paying. Not much out of the ordinary happened there but that was what made it feel relatively safe. I did try the pub at the bottom of the hill once with James, but the crowds and the paranoia made that a deeply uncomfortable experience. Paranoia was something that the German had emphatically assured me I did not have. To me though, it was very real. Going out began to edge me back to some form of reality.

My contact with those I'd known so well began to fall off though. Becky and Sophie, Steve and Neil, and many of the other musical brethren remained fairly constant in their contact. Trapper too was still a constant in my life. But news from the Cambridge guys became more and more sporadic. My old tutor Chris kept in quite regular touch and I continued to visit from time to time. As the news of the others waned, I began to get disturbed. The belief that they didn't want to talk to me gripped me more strongly as the months went by. That then began to feed into the illness. Another paradox cropped up: I felt they didn't want to talk to me so I didn't call. They in turn failed to keep up with me, partly because they didn't know what to say, and partly because they thought I didn't want any contact. I yearned to hear from them, much as I did with Rachel, yet I feared that phone ringing. No one seemed prepared to take the initiative. With that came paranoia and paranoia fed on paranoia.

As my outside contacts started to wane, chance appeared again. I had been searching around for some time for another route out. There appeared to be no hope with the Mental Health System, they just seemed to be bankrupt of ideas. Things were happening there but, as yet, I was being kept in the dark. For some time the only person I felt was helping me and was on my side was my GP. On more than one occasion he had allowed me in at no notice at all because the burdens of illness were too great. He had also been searching around for answers with only limited success but at least he listened to me, and more importantly, believed me. There can't be too many GPs surgeries that have hypnotherapists working with them, but as chance would have it, mine had one who started that summer. It was at one of our weekly meetings that the Doctor mentioned him and asked if I wanted to give it a go. My mind immediately raced off exploring the possibilities. Would it work? It's a load of bullshit! What have I got to lose? Maybe there's hope. But I was just so desperate I was prepared to give anything a go, even if I had to pay for it. Meagre though my resources were, I was able to get some help from my parents for it. Ultimately I had nothing to lose at all. My agreement followed almost immediately and an appointment was made for the following week.

When I met him, he was a complete surprise. He was much older than I had anticipated, a big man with almost white hair. He was softly spoken and made me feel most welcome. He was, in fact, a retired GP who had moved into hypnotherapy late in his career. The fact that he was a Doctor did not really put me off because his manner was so different from what I had been used to in the last couple of years. He really gave off the impression that not only did he care, but he also intended to work for me, for my benefit. That seemed to be his main motive despite the fact that it was a private treatment. Money just seemed incidental. That may have been naive of me, but it didn't really matter. He was calm and not judgmental as we talked before treatment. I had no real idea or expectation of the treatment, it was just a new path to be trodden, and it really couldn't be much worse than what I had had before. I found myself at complete ease purely by his manner.

Being hypnotised when it happened was a most odd experience. I found myself aware but not aware. I was utterly focused yet confused as well. I also found myself vaguely wondering if I was supposed to feel something else. It was completely unlike what I had experienced watching at a May Ball some years before. I was awake but in a different place. I remember being aware of what I was saying to him but unable to stop even if I'd wanted to. But I didn't feel the need to. There were no inhibitions here, he didn't have the power to put me back in the Palace. What I seemed to be saying was little different to what I had been saying all along but there was no longer the need to be so guarded in my responses. It was just very relaxing and unthreatening. He brought me round after a period of time that I was completely unable to determine. Time seemed to have stood still and looking at my watch made little difference. Still wondering whether it was real or not, or whether I had done it properly, we talked again.

A Pillar of Impotence

He seemed very disturbed by what I had told him. It suddenly dawned on me that he had seen into my madness in a way that no one else had. He trusted completely his observations and saw how gravely ill I was. He seemed to see my pain and accept it as the truth. No one else except my GP had done that. It was a new angle but my instinct told me that maybe he could help me. And that was completely new to me. I didn't know where it would lead me but I knew I had to take that path. Finding someone with just a little insight was new. He seemed to be with me not against as the so called experts seemed to be. I wasn't expecting any miracles but I felt a tiny modicum of hope. And any real hope had been way beyond my consciousness since it had all started. We arranged to meet again in a week, then the week after, and then again. Each week a little more leaked out and he gained a greater understanding. He realised how vulnerable and out of control my mind was, and he backed me. A new path was set, again by chance.

It would not be long though before the old and the new paths would collide. One of the things that had always annoyed me about the professionals was that there always seemed to be a hidden agenda. That agenda seemed to be paramount, and as one would expect, I took no part in it. Things started to unravel rather innocuously. It must have been at the height of summer when I went along to one of my regular sessions with the German. I'd been going to see her for about eighteen months at that stage and I was still trying to work out exactly what it was about; there seemed to me to have been no discernible change in that time, at least not as a result of that. It was a day no different from any other, and I wasn't expecting it to be any different to any other session. I walked in, sat down, and waited for her to start her research. It was her opening comment that threw me off balance.

"I think we've got as much out of this as we are going to get so we'll only have two more sessions after this week." I wasn't quite sure what to make of that but just let her continue. "I think you've improved over these past few months."

"How have I done that?" There was no way that I could see that the past year and a half had made any difference to me. I was maybe sleeping a bit better. The after effects of the overdose had passed. But nothing had been resolved; I was still living in my own private hell just wanting to die every time I went to sleep. Death was still the obsession and suicidal thoughts swept over me many times a day. My head was still pounding and her voice kept on quietly echoing around that same head. Nothing of any significance had changed since the start.

"You've stopped intellectualising as much as you did."

"So what? What exactly does that mean?" None of what she was saying had any bearing on what passed for my reality. She just went on with her research. I didn't feel any more enlightened than I had been three years before.

The session passed without further incident and I just went home wondering what was going to happen next. She didn't appear to have any idea what we were going to do once the next two appointments were finished. But she was playing it very close to her chest. Things were afoot, but it was not deemed necessary that I should know the plan or their findings yet; I would have to wait another month to find that out. Two weeks later my dalliance with Cognitive Behavioural Therapy was over. I still sought answers in my head as to what precisely therapy had been all about.

Whilst still in my confusion about therapy, a brown envelope dropped through my letter box. Fear gripped me as it did all the others I knew when such an event happened. Too frightened to open it, I left it on my desk amongst piles of other paperwork. As long as it was on the top I would know it was there. A couple of days later, I gingerly opened it to find a map and another of those standard forms requiring me to attend a medical examination at Canterbury the following week. There was no explanation as to why I had been singled out, or as to the letter's timing. I had had no previous correspondence from the DHSS that related to this. There was just a message in bold letters telling me that "If you do not attend it may affect your benefits." The fear deepened instantly. Things had been a little easier since things had been sorted out. I didn't have much at all and now it appeared that they could take away what little I had. I was mobile only because my parents paid for the car; that was an extreme blessing. Bemused by this, I started to ask around to see if any of the others had had similar letters. None had. Why was I being singled out? Like most things in my life it didn't make sense. But I knew that I had no choice. My Doctor had faithfully filled out a form once a month to sign me off sick; now they seemed to doubt his judgement. What I feared most was that they would tell me I had to look for work. The sense of persecution returned in all its terrible splendour.

John came with me as I set out for what could be, in my eyes, another cataclysmic meeting. It was hot and difficult to park. Canterbury had always a difficult place to park, and now I found myself in a Resident's Permit Zone. This was new to me and I could feel the tension and stress rising as the fear of a parking fine loomed large in my mind. We hurried into the building to be given a parking permit. Back to the car we went then returned to face whatever destiny awaited me. Sitting there was akin to a cross between waiting for the dentist and fearing one's driving test. It was warm and stuffy adding to my frayed nerves. Then I was called into a room in a very formal way and found myself confronted by an elderly Doctor. His manner was gruff and equally formal. An endless stream of questions followed most of which seemed to be about my physical health. I told my story as best I could but it just didn't seem to fit his remit. Whoever had designed this test had clearly not had mental illness or disability in mind; it just didn't relate at all to my condition. At the end he checked my heart and blood pressure telling me that although it had no bearing on my illness, the test required him to do it. With that he let me go. It seemed to have gone on an eternity but when I checked my watch, it had taken just over half an hour. That half an hour was one of the worse I had experienced since my madness started. I was there to be judged and there was nothing I could do about it. And it was all for the sake of about £15 per week. There was a sense of relief when I emerged back into the waiting room to find John quietly reading a magazine, but it was tainted by the knowledge that I now had to wait for an undisclosed length of time before my fate and judgement were sealed. A Doctor whom I never met before held my meagre financial situation in his hands. I would never see him again, and he had no idea what damage his verdict could do. I left feeling that I had been put on trial and still wondering what that verdict would be; judgement would be adjourned until he saw fit to do so. In the meantime, I just had to wait.

It was a Saturday when I received that verdict. As usual, it was delivered by brown envelope. It had taken only just under a week. Frightened though I was, I knew I couldn't wait this time and I opened it immediately. Inside I found another standard form explaining that I had recently attended a medical examination and that the results were written below. In the space provided was a message scrawled in what looked like the hand of a young child who had yet to master the art of writing. "You are only 50% disabled and therefore need less money." My mind instantly exploded into another myriad of thoughts each jostling for prominence. Shit! Fuck! Why me? Less money. I'm already living on a pittance. Who was he? How can you define a disability in percentage terms? That's just not possible. On and on they went but above all it was the sense of persecution that won out. Panic set in. How was I going to manage on so little? I lived to travel and now they seemed to be taking that away from me. Why, why, why? Nothing could console me that weekend. All I could do was to appeal and that meant going in to see them at the office, but that would have to wait until Monday. Then came all the normal feelings again. Despair. Anger. The voice. And, blotting all else out, suicide.

The Folkestone branch of the DHSS is one of the most depressing buildings that I've ever had the misfortune to visit. It lies in a large complex of buildings, each interlinked, and built of red brick, probably in the early to mid 1970s. I had had to go there as a regularly biweekly visitor before they signed me off. I had not been there in about eighteen months and thanked good fortune most days that that experience was over as a normal occurrence. On that fateful Monday morning I found myself waiting patiently for my ticket number to come up. Around me were many desperate and angry people. The staff, peering out from behind their glass screens, were manfully, patiently, and fearfully doing their jobs. I had always had some sympathy for them for doing such a thankless job, but at the same time, they were the enemy. They had power that I feared, just like the shrinks. At least though, it was not the power to put me back in the Palace. I trembled normally, but that day I was shaking with fear as well. I yearned for nicotine but all around me were notices telling me I could not smoke. Others ignored them and the security guards outside seemed to take no notice. Not me though; as ever, I abided by the rules. I didn't really heed the motives of those around; they were just as desperate as I was. Or at least, they had to give that appearance for their turn at what the Americans would call a booth. I've never really worked out what we would call it.

My number came up and I slowly moved toward the window, body shaking and heart and head pounding. It was a young woman behind the glass, young but older than me. She seemed friendly as I explained my story and handed over to her the form with the scrawl on it, telling her as I did so that I wanted to appeal the decision.

"The form is wrong, you get the same amount of money but it's a different benefit. You're just moving from Severe Disablement Allowance to Income Support."

"I still want to appeal."

"There's no point" she carried on, "it's still the same amount of money." But she'd missed my point. I knew quite how debilitating my condition was and I wanted that recognised. Try as I might, the message didn't get through. It didn't and I found myself giving up in the end. I left feeling slightly relieved but wondering why I had been put through so much more trauma just for the sake of a different benefit.

There is a curious quirk to the British benefit system that some people get a Christmas bonus of £10. They tell me that the amount has been the same for decades but when one lives on around £50 per week, that makes a great deal of difference. Old Age Pensioners get it. So do those on Severe Disablement Allowance. Those on Income Support do not. That Christmas, I lost out again.

I had long ago formulated a theory that I called *The Right Illness Theory*. My theory ran along the lines that the treatment one received as a psychiatric patient was directly proportional to the severity of the diagnosis one was given. The result of which was that people given extreme diagnoses such as schizophrenia and manic depression were treated far more seriously than those with apparently more mundane diagnoses such as depression and anxiety. It was not a case of correct diagnosis, although I had long suspected that mine was incorrect. I truly believed that I had a psychotic illness but nobody seemed to want to do anything about it. I also had suspicions that the role of the key worker differed dependent on diagnosis, but I was never proved right or wrong on that. I seemed to be lumbered with an OT as a key worker, my friends with the appropriate psychotic diagnoses, with the one exception of Matt, all had Psychiatric Nurses. My experience at the hands of the DHSS appeared to correlate to the theory; I never knew anyone with a psychotic diagnosis to be called for a medical. For years I was the only one. I had survived another battle with them; there would be more in the future.

The first public appearance of parts of what had been the hidden agenda became known soon after. My relationship with Vicky, so badly jeopardised at the start, had now descended into farce. There now existed an open hatred between us, she wanted to get rid of me, and I wanted to get rid of her just as badly. Yet she was still in control, and I was as powerless as ever. So it was for my second visit to the consultant. I don't recall the German being there or ever seeing her again, but the visit followed the previous pattern. He talked almost exclusively to Vicky and when he did turn to speak to me he took me completely by surprise.

"I think we should work towards discharging you in three months. We'll meet again then and formalise the discharge." The only other thing he said was that he wanted me to go out and do something I'd never done before. That didn't seem to make sense. But then again, neither did the rest of it.

I left in a very confused and slightly frightened state. I couldn't believe that they were going to stop what little support they gave me for no apparent reason. Maybe it was a test. What was clear was that within three months I would be back on my own again, and, as far as I felt, no better in measurable terms than I'd been at the start. Now they just seemed to want to cast me asunder and wash their hands of me. They had never really been able to do much to get me better but having something was better than having nothing. And that was a feeling that we all to shared. Most of us felt outcast by society and the stigma it attached to us. Now the very people who were supposed to care and help us seemed intent on making me an outcast as well. I pondered what to do but no answers came.

As the weeks slipped by my fear grew. Autumn had always been marginally better for me, primarily because of my passion for the American sport that started at that time. Not now. All I could see was the same black hole that I had descended into three years before. I had slithered up out of it an infinitesimal amount over time. Now I could feel my tenuous grasp loosening again. The plunge back down began to fill my waking thoughts along with all the other usual thoughts. Three months is a short time if one is frightened. The sense of impending doom was accompanied by thoughts of death, the volume of the calls and desires increasing daily. What no one had told me was that there was another part to the hidden agenda. I would have to wait for that as the last vestiges of summer disappeared and the leaves fell. With that came a grim October.

Chapter 16

Secrets Exposed

I don't really recall exactly when I started to read again. My fall from the heady days of Cambridge had been precipitous, and reading and understanding intellectual literature had served as a kind of tape measure for my illness. The first two years had been very easy: have a tutorial once a week; get a reading list and an essay title; then just do it. I had it down to the fine art of reading for three hours per weeks, then writing for a further three. Skim reading was essential, as was the need to pick out what was important, then do the bare minimum. That left time for everything else. The third year was harder, partly due to a greater degree of timetabled work, but mainly because I was already very ill. But I managed, including the huge volume of often dull medieval work that was deemed vital to passing. All that went when I left.

For many months I could barely read a word. When I did start, gingerly and secretly, it was always short and simple work. I couldn't read anything of the level that I had had to do before. The greatest handicap was a chronic inability to retain information; it just went in then straight out again. This led to frustration, which, in turn, fed back into the illness and my mood.

That mood, always low and unpredictable, was accompanied and dominated by death and the desire to die. That had been the be all and end all of my existence since the day before my graduation in 1991. It was perhaps a natural extension of that feeling that led me to True Crime books when I finally began to read more substantially. Many an hour was spent in bookshops, almost always bargain book shops, rooting out anything I could find on death. I think the first book that I got was Gordon Burn's biography of Peter Sutcliffe, *Somebody's Husband, Somebody's Son.* This, however, proved to be far too hard a read for me and it was left undisturbed on my bookshelf for a number of years after. Other things were easier, and, by the time I went to Cadiz, I was reading again if rather slowly. The crimes were often horrific, but what attracted me was what exactly was going on in the minds of these people. Of course, I, like everyone else, could never hope, or perhaps want, to know what that was. But I was undeterred and it filled in some more of my interminable days. Although one could hardly describe such reading as light, in comparison to what I was used to, it was both that and manageable. It would take many more years before I even attempted, at least beyond the first page or two, anything beyond this genre. It was against this background and my obsession with death, that the storm that had been silently gathering around me emerged in the autumn of 1993.

In the weeks immediately following the ultimatum I spent a great deal of time talking with those afflicted with illness about what was happening to me. Almost all of them were shocked, confused and above all, fearful that the same would happen to them. Many spoke to their key workers about it. This was taken by them and then relayed back to me that I was manipulating others and putting their health and safety in jeopardy. It was accusation that both appalled and angered me. Not only was it not true, it was also offensive. But manipulation on my part, or a perception of it, was very much part of their thinking; they just never mentioned it to me. In fact, that was an aspect of their thinking that I would only be aware of long after my first partial recovery. As it was then, it merely added to the downward spiral.

My friends were not the only ones to be alarmed by my rapid mental descent. The deterioration of my condition was quickly picked up by the hypnotherapist. He was so concerned that he immediately wrote to the consultant expressing his view that my suicidal feelings and urges would soon be beyond my control, and that I needed to be seen straight away and be allowed to stay. The response was a terse letter, not from the consultant, but from Vicky telling him in no uncertain terms that it was inappropriate that I should be seeing a hypnotherapist and that he should leave it to them. He described it me as the "rudest letter I have received in over forty years in the medical profession." And that was from an OT. I didn't see him much after that. Perhaps I was foolish.

It was a Thursday when I finally collapsed again mentally. For weeks the pressure had been building. The deadline was still about two weeks away, but breaking point came early. Thursday afternoon was always the social afternoon at the Day Service. I sat there alone with my thoughts. They were spinning away on their own and no intervention or contact slowed my mind down. I was just in free fall. I had always kept the worse of my mental state to myself when with my parents. Partly I felt I had to do it because my mind was mine alone, but also to protect them from what they almost certainly they would not be able to handle. But as I got home, I could no longer contain things. I sat cross legged on the bed rocking back and forth murmuring to myself. My mum came in and I finally managed to force something out.

"I think I'm breaking down again." That was all I could manage. Realising how bad things were, they immediately called the GP. Whether he came to me or I went to him is blotted out of my memory. Whatever happened, I found myself waiting to see the consultant early the following week. Memories of that weekend are no longer with me, but it would have been terrible. The problem that I faced though was to get him to talk to me and not to her. I also needed someone to be with me to fight for me against people who were now a roundly hated enemy. Help was at hand however.

I first met Heather and Chris at the MIND meetings on Wednesday nights. I didn't know them too well but they seemed very caring, and ran the group, along with others, very well. It would be some time before I realised it, but they were, in fact, Matt's parents. They were also formidable advocates and campaigners for the rights of the mentally ill. It also helped that Heather worked at the hospital and was well known there. Heather had clout, and she was prepared to use it for me. She had a tough reputation for helping the ill and as such was a feared opponent for the egos of the professionals. On the whole, they didn't like dealing with her.

It was late in the afternoon when we arrived and sat down in the small waiting area. We came with a three part agenda: to stop the discharge; to get rid of Vicky as my key worker; and to get a definitive diagnosis from him. Their agenda was still largely unknown. What we walked into though was an immediate impasse. I refused to see him with Vicky present, he in turn refused that. He insisted that Heather did not come in with me. I was equally adamant that I wasn't seeing anyone without her. Tensions rose as we sat there and they came back and forth trying to negotiate. But buoyed by having someone to finally fight for me, we stuck to our ground and they conceded. The first small but significant victory.

He was a different man this time. Backed into a corner he had no choice but to talk to me rather than to others. After much deliberation and argument he acceded to the getting rid of Vicky and to letting me stay. He would not be drawn on diagnosis however much we pushed. There was more though.

"I want to send you for some different treatment in London." There was a pause before he continued. "I don't think you are going to find it easy."

What a strange thing to say, I thought, doesn't he think this is hard enough already? I had a mixed sense of relief that they'd not abandoned me, but also of curiosity. He seemed to be accepting that I was very ill but going into the unknown was frightening. But the breakthrough outweighed the fear, at least initially.

"But first I want you to go and see another Doctor in Ashford." What could that mean? Unsure we carried on with the conversation for a while. After that he let Heather go and asked me a series of what seemed inane questions. Then the meeting was over.

We'd achieved most of what we had wanted and there seemed to be a way forward. I wondered about this other Doctor and why that was deemed necessary. It never occurred to me that he was seeking a second opinion. But then again, how could I conceive of that when he had no apparent opinion in the first place? I was disappointed that he was incapable of giving me a diagnosis, but my mood did lift with the relief that I still had some contact and I no longer had Vicky controlling my life. I also learned the life long lesson that in the Mental Health System, it always paid off to have an advocate.

It was a warm autumn day when I stepped off the train at what would soon be known as Ashford International station. Ashford had always been a place that I loathed but times were changing there with coming of the Channel Tunnel and the commerce that that would bring. To this day the thought of Ashford as a base for international travel seems ludicrous to me and to many of the locals. Even they often referred to the place as Trashford. Ashford town centre is surrounded by a wide and usually congested ring road. The base of the local Community Mental Health Team lies on that road, but a short walk from the terminus.

I was alone when I went up there, intrigued and baffled by what might take place there. The building proved easy to find, and, having introduced myself and announcing my appointment, I sat down to wait. It was a ritual that I had to follow with alarming regularity. That day it was but a short wait before a youngish man called me into his office. He appeared much friendlier than any of the previous incarnations of psychiatry I'd met. He was very good at putting me at ease. Despite that, I was still suspicious. The ice-breaker though was that he was a Cambridge man. And that was the way in.

Time passed quickly as we talked at length on many things, but the focus usually revolved around childhood and Cambridge. Like the German, he was of course researching but the conversation was less stilted and he took a far greater part in the proceedings than she had. As we spoke I was naively unaware of two key factors, firstly that he had supervised the original Cognitive Behavioural Therapy, and secondly that he was aiming for a predetermined conclusion. As a historian it is always a great trap to try to fit the evidence to a preconceived theory or notion. Better to hear the evidence then decide what happened than to do it the other way round. Maybe psychiatry is different but that was precisely what he was doing. Pick up what you can and let it fit.

I spent a good two hours with him before he wearily announced that he needed to mull over his thoughts for a while. We arranged to meet again in two weeks time to talk some more and then see where that led. Moderately buoyed by a wholly new experience of psychiatry, I caught the train home and waited.

The next meeting was shorter and started in the more or less the same way. After a while he stopped to speak. Here was the wisdom of an expert, in goes the information, turn the handle and out churns the answer.

"I don't think you have depression at all." Those words made me take notice. "I think you have a Narcissistic Personality Disorder."

What the fuck is that was my first thought but it came out in a milder way.

"What's that?" Anything was better than to be told I was depressed but I knew what narcissism was and it didn't sound too good.

Then he said something very odd: "That doesn't mean you are a psychopath." Why would I think that? He went on to give a lengthy but baffling description of what it was using some story of a man who sold furniture but believed he was some great dealer. It seemed to all revolve around some form of delusion. It all sounded very well but something was unnerving and obviously wrong with what he was saying. All the things that I had done in the past that we had talked at such length about were true. Everything was related as it had happened. Nothing in what I had said had differed from the talk in the early days. The only difference now was that I did actually talk about hearing Rachel's voice. He had seized upon that but apparently dismissed it.

The next stage was to arrange an appointment to see a man in London to find out if I was suitable for treatment and then proceed from there. That would take time. I have never seen the man in Ashford since but his name is one I often hear and one I would, in time, learn to bitterly regret ever hearing. There was a curious mix of feelings in my mind as I sat on the train back. It was a step in my eyes to lose the label of depression. On the other hand the new diagnosis didn't seem to make any sense. Not only did I not understand what it was, there were also clear flaws. I would have to wait some time before I realised the diagnosis of Personality Disorder was infinitely worse than depression. I was unaware that I had now been placed in the last box available; and that ultimately meant being written off. I was no longer considered to be ill, it was just me that was wrong. It was only really Heather who realised how bad this new development was. But she kept her counsel. Privately she was stunned and disturbed by it. She was also adamant that they were completely wrong.

It was whilst waiting for my trip to London that chance was to take me down another path. Although we lived in the same house, my parents and I lived essentially different lives. My dad was still away in Scotland much of the time but visited regularly. They were just as exasperated by the lack of progress made as I was and were looking for anything that could help. It had been some time before that my mum had taken up Japanese lessons for fun at the local Adult Education centre. She had apparently committed a terrible faux pas early on. In very simple terms the class were asking each other questions and getting answers in equally simple terms. She was asked "how is your son?" to which she replied that I wasn't very well and left it at that. The tutor then told them that in Japan nobody talked about being unwell and such things were usually glossed over. Mother and tutor became firm friends after that and the lady from Japan gave a way forward.

I had never heard of Rudolph Steiner until he was mentioned to me by my mother. There was apparently a Steiner school on the outskirts of the very town which played host to the Archbishop's Palace. Yukino's children went there along with the children of a Doctor near Maidstone. And he ran a Steiner treatment centre in the grounds of the old asylum at Barming. It was a strange coincidence that in the two locations which I knew of, Steiner was accompanied by an asylum. It had been some time in the offing, but they had made contact with him and arranged for me to meet him. When they told me I could see no reason not to go. Maybe he could help.

It was cold and early on a Saturday morning when we got in the car to go to meet him. We arrived to find a beautiful modern building set against a backdrop of this huge derelict asylum. It was equally beautiful but far more menacing. Like the asylum, the new building seemed deserted. It was also locked. We wandered about for a while looking for a way to get in but found no joy. Just as we were thinking of leaving, a tall, slightly dishevelled figure appeared apologising profusely for his tardiness. He opened the building and led me into a small consulting room. This was David.

"Do want your parents to be present?" was his opening line.
"No way" came my immediate response. Then I told him my story. It was the utter compassion and conviction that he displayed that captivated me. I was, on the whole, very distrustful of the medical profession but he was different to so many I'd met. He listened, spoke, believed and cared. He was concerned about the level of medication which, although modest in comparison to my daily doses of the pink pills, still had a profound effect on my ability to function. But above all else, he seemed to have some understanding

of the illness itself. That was new. I told him of the proposed treatment in London and he said that he knew the man I was going to see. He reassured me that he was a highly intelligent man who could really help. Nevertheless, he felt he could help in the meantime.

What he proposed was that I should come up there once a week to see an Art Therapist initially. That struck me as odd but interesting; the previous suggestion of that had been dismissed out of hand without consultation. He also proposed that due to the distance I needed to travel and the tiredness that driving always induced in me, I should come up the night before and stay at his house. I could then see the therapist and travel home afterwards. I agreed and we struck the deal. As we drove back there was just a hint of belief in my mind. I'd found something different, and as with the hypnotherapist, some hope. But in the light of that previous experience, I resolved to keep this secret. I wasn't going to let anyone fuck this up for me. This was mine, my own hidden agenda.

With them blissfully unaware of my new direction, I carried on at the Day Service. There was a bit of an air of suspicion amongst some of the staff and it was very apparent that Vicky was not overly happy with the way that things had turned out but that was tempered by the fact that she didn't really have to work with me in any meaningful way. I was given a new key worker, or as it transpired, he had inherited me. He told me in our first one to one session that at the team meeting there had been a deafening silence amongst them when the issue had been raised as to who would take over. He had stepped into the breech. Tom had been the new co-ordinator of the place for only a few months. The previous incumbent of the post had been a man whom I'd got on with very well, and, unlike most of the rest of them, I respected him for his honesty and compassion. It made no difference to me whether I worked with a man or a woman, what did make a difference was that he was experienced, wiser, and infinitely more pragmatic. He was no young crusader. It proved to be a good fit. As we waited for the meeting in London we talked some about this magical new diagnosis. But it didn't seem to make me any wiser, nor did it quell my doubts about it.

The initial wait to go to London was neither long nor eventful. I had no real qualms about meeting the man himself, my only worry was overcoming my appalling sense of direction that had developed with my illness. Going to new places troubled me intensely. This was a function of just how much I had lost my capacity to remember things. I was not very familiar with London, my knowledge being confined more or less to how to get from Charing Cross to Liverpool Street on my occasional trips to Cambridge, and that only required getting on the Circle Line of the tube. Above ground was another story. Everything looked the same there. However, the journey this day was a short and relatively easy one. With the directions given to me, my destination was but a short walk to the left outside the station. I found a rather decrepit and nondescript building set back a little way from the main road behind a pub. It seemed to date from maybe just after the war, about four stories high with a strange looking metal cage on the roof. There had been no access to the roof at the Palace so no need for it. But this was another nuthouse and there was a need here. It struck me as being a potentially very dark place, shadowed for much of the day by its surroundings. There was however, a time in the late morning where the little courtyard outside was bathed in sunlight. It was at that time that I arrived. Despite the light it was cold and crisp that December morning.

On entering I was asked to sit down to wait for the great man. It was not long before an older and rather distinguished looking man emerged from a small office right by the front door and asked me to come in. The first thing that struck me was how easy going and friendly he was; first impressions would, in time, prove to be deceptive. We'd only been talking for a very short space of time when the phone on his desk rang.

"Would you excuse please, I've been waiting for this call for some time." His expression was effortless and he spoke in what older people would have called a jolly way. He was all smiles and good humour, eloquent and disarming. And I was lulled by the charm.

His call over, we reverted to our conversation. David had been right about this man, his intellect was obvious. He was also unlike any shrink I had met before. It was just like having a normal, intelligent conversation. We talked a great deal of Rachel and of Cambridge. A chance remark took us into jumbled world of choral scholarships, Cambridge entrance, and the horse trading that always goes on behind the scene. Much had been explained to me at the time and this I recounted to him exactly as it was told to me. Back and forth we went, both apparently surprising the other on occasion. What he didn't let on then was that I came with a reputation, one passed on by those back in Kent. And that had already clouded his judgement.

It seemed to have only lasted a few minutes before he gave forth his proposal. In fact we had been in there for over an hour but time had gone quickly.

"I think we can help you. Will you excuse me again while I make the arrangements?" With that he picked up the phone to arrange a date for me to come and see the unit itself. He explained a little about how the set up worked and the various therapies they used. Yet again art therapy was one all people did, reinforcing my feeling of how strange it had been to have had that idea dismissed earlier. Much of what he said made little impact but what did stick was his comment that they treated many more women than men. It didn't seem particularly odd, but for some reason it stayed with me. With an arrangement to come back the following week, to be there at what seemed the impossible time to arrive of 9.30, I headed back for the train. I was suitably impressed; this was a wholly new, and very different world. It smacked of professionalism, a far cry from what had passed for the norm over the last two years.

I made it with but a few minutes to spare having run down from the station. I was tired and cold and a bit bewildered. I was ushered into a room full of people and sat in someone's seat. Moving on I found somewhere else to perch. There was great tension, fear and anticipation in the room. Anxiety and nervousness was etched over the faces of almost everyone in there. When the door closed, many were sitting on the floor. I was asked to introduce myself which in did by standing and giving perhaps more information than anyone expected. Round the room each person gave their name, some quietly and shyly, others more audibly and with confidence. The room was alive with undercurrents and a sense of dread. But there was silence. We just sat there. I wondered what was supposed to happen next. Still nothing. After a while I glanced at my watch as surreptitiously as I could. It was 9.50. We'd been there for twenty minutes and nothing had happened. Then it started. A barbed comment, then a few more. Then the first sign of a defence; or was it defiance? Within minutes the room was buzzing with verbal bile directed at one person. She held her own. As an observer it was both amazing and unnerving. Time had changed in that place, its pace defined in sections, slow silence then rapid fury. In no time, it was over. It was only then that relief and calm returned; the tension was gone.

I spent the rest of the day talking to both staff and patients. Lunch was good and everyone seemed on the surface to get on quite well. But still there was a sense of the hidden. There was a lot more laughter than I had seen in such a place before. People came and went to and fro their various groups during the day, and they went out. That was different. It didn't have the air of oppression that had accompanied my stay at the Palace. It was much freer here.

I came away with mixed feelings. It had been a good day but there was the prospect of that intense bile flying around in that first group. When I went there I knew I'd have to endure that every day, and maybe at some stage, be the target. They warned me that there was a lengthy list of people before me in the queue and that it could take many months to get there. There was also the unspoken feeling that this was the last and only chance for me and my condition. As with everything else in Mental Health, options are portrayed as choices, but the choices were clearly loaded. All I could do now was wait. And while I waited I had the legacy of Rudolph Steiner.

Throughout the winter I made the drive to Barming once a week. Staying made life easier for me, but throughout that time I always felt guilty for intruding. Their approach was entirely new to me. They worked with me to try to rebuild what was left of my broken mind. They didn't care for diagnosis or hold any preconceptions about their patients. Art was one of those subjects that had passed me by. It wasn't that I didn't like it or work at it, it was just that something had to give to make way for all the music. And art was the chosen area. I'd never really been taught anything. I found I actually quite liked what Hazel taught me. Unusually for me it didn't concern me as to whether or not I was good at it, I just did it for the sake of it. I did wonder where exactly it was leading and what I was supposed to get out of it but that was a secondary thought. The whole place exuded a wonderful sense of calm. This calm was tempered by the ominous presence of the asylum in the background, a feeling I never really overcame. But I felt comfortable there, and no one judged me.

There was one other glorious thing that happened that winter. The Archbishop's Palace was closed for good. That cheered and relieved me. With that, a new unit was opened in Ashford. It proved in time to be little better.

I'd been going to Barming for a couple of months when David gingerly asked if I'd like to see a counsellor as well. He was reluctant to do this as he felt that I'd done so much talking already that I might not want to do any more, but he felt that it could be useful. My agreement led to what would prove to be a significant discovery, but the magnitude of that discovery would not be clear until many years later. Bons was Dutch. We talked each week in a very relaxing way and she gradually built up what would prove to be a remarkably accurate picture of me.

The year ended in much the same fashion as the previous few. I was very low and erratic in my mood. Rachel was still pounding away in my mind and the headaches continued. Suicide was an eternal theme. Flashbacks continued to plague me. The Day Service was still the Day Service. I was waiting for change. I was confused even with the new treatment in my life. In the East war continued with added barbarity. The names of previously obscure town littered our news outlets and the term "ethnic cleansing" was now clearly installed in the English language; it was about to hit Africa too. To the West the flames of Waco had died out but not its legacy. Hell was all around and I was still in my private hell.

It was early in the New Year that Bons inadvertently made her breakthrough. We were talking one afternoon when she tried to conceptualise what life was like for me.

"It sounds to me as though you live in an underground lift. Ground level is being well but you never get there. The lift merely moves up and down at random and you have no control over it."

Brilliant I thought. Someone has finally understood what it was like. The description was astoundingly accurate. I rejoiced that someone could describe my life with its twists and unexpected turns. I had never changed my story from day one. It had always been like having a light switch in my head, and that light switch was turned on at random. Life was shit all the time, but once the switch moved, it just got infinitely worse. It had always been like that but none of them attached any significance to it. Pleased though I was, I still didn't know where we went from there; or how helpful it would be.

January turned to February and still the waiting went on.

Chapter 17

The Hotel California

I have no personal reason to remember the date 24th February 1994; it simply wasn't one of my dates. I do know that my mood would have been low. I would certainly have felt suicidal. Likewise, I would have heard Rachel's voice. I would have gone to bed that night after taking my pills, little blue and white capsules now, and wanted not to wake up the next day. These were the norms for me, the everyday occurrences of my existence. I would, with hindsight, speculate that I may have been in one of my more stable periods. The books tell me that in certain parts of the country, it was a cold and grim day; I have no doubt that that was true, and no reason to believe that it was any different in Kent. It was, after all, February.

That was the day that police went to an obscure and scruffy address in Gloucester looking for a body; in the weeks to come they would unearth a graveyard. An equally obscure builder and his plump wife would very quickly become the most talked about people in the country, and not long after, in much of the world. It started slowly in the press but my interest was pricked very quickly. With each passing day the headlines became more lurid and the speculation more intense. This was tabloid gold dust, each one trying to out do the others. People's ghoulish side took centre stage, and jokes about a man called Fred were everywhere. I scoured every paper I could get my hands on as it was a subject I spent a great deal of time reading about. The horror of the daily pictures was often lost in those headlines and people just wanted more and more detail. It just seemed to get worse as the weeks of the end of winter went by. This was the backdrop to my wait to go to London.

It was on a Friday, just after lunch, at the end of March that the call came. Unusually for me, given my fear of phones, I answered the call. It was a man's voice, a man clearly older than me. He told me that a place was now available and asked if I'd like to take it. He was most insistent that if I was to take it, I had to go the very next day. I was reluctant to go that quickly merely because I was due to attend a funeral on the Monday after the weekend. I'd known her vaguely at the Day Service but I felt quite strongly that I should go.

She'd died of natural causes. I had yet to experience the traumas of a successful suicide; mine had been singularly unsuccessful. It pissed me off that I would be prevented from going but it was clear that I had little choice. It was a choice like all others in mental health, a loaded one. I was of course oblivious to the chronic shortage of beds in London. So I agreed to go the following morning.

It was about lunchtime when I got to London. Laden with suitcase and bag I sat down alone with my thoughts at the station. I wasn't really sure where I was going or what I was doing. I had no idea where this new course would take me but it was clear that it was probably the last chance. Part of me wanted to feel in the elite of nutters; that was a sentiment that many of us were to feel. Most of the time it was just a way to alleviate the pressure. I was alone with my thoughts, people passing nonchalantly by. In London I was just another nobody, an anonymous face in an anonymous crowd. On reflection after the experience, that feeling proved to be largely correct. Thoughts collected I headed down the road for the short walk to what would be my home for the foreseeable future.

It was quite quiet when I got there, many people having gone home for the weekend. There were no therapy sessions at weekends but the day proved rather bewildering with what seemed to be an endless stream of meetings with Doctors and other staff. For those who have known me for a while, it is hard for them to remember what I was like when they first met me. For all the confidence they perceived me to show they forget just how quiet and shy I am around those I don't know. It has always been such, constantly trying to work others out before becoming more out going. It was just the same at the ward. It helped though that another new patient arrived on the same day. She, like the rest of them appeared friendly. Some of the other faces were familiar in a limited way from my previous visit. There was a new face though, a young women who was very ill. She had, it transpired, been brought in for the weekend because she was having a very difficult time. She was due to be discharged after the weekend and that would provide the first major drama of my stay.

There was, however, a more immediate problem though. It had been stressed very strongly at my previous visit that I shouldn't bring any pills with me. Unaware when I was going to go to London

A Pillar of Impotence

I had collected my medication from the chemist earlier that week. There was a month's supply of the blue and white capsules sitting on my bedside table back in Kent but none in London. In one of my first meetings there they had brought up the issue of my pills. It seemed that I was on an unusually low dose, one that was not considered to be a "therapeutic" dose. Therefore they proposed that they would increase it fairly quickly. I had no opinion either way. No anti-depressant had ever had an anti-depressant effect on me. I had been on at least six different types over the years but to no avail. This logically suggested to me that maybe they were wrong but no one was interested in my opinion. What they did though was make me sleep, and, for that very reason, were priceless to me. The blue and white capsules had a major sedative effect as a side effect; and that was why I took them. When it came to the first evening I was informed that they didn't have any in stock. They then enquired if I had brought any with me. The first crack appeared at that point. Don't trust, don't trust. The thought echoed around my mind. Predictably enough my sleep was very limited that first weekend. It was not the last that would be heard about the blue and white relief.

On the Sunday the pace quickened. Before the others had started to arrive back I was told my presence was required for an emergency group. Baffled as to what that was all about I sat there mystified as a woman I had met previously started to talk. I was immediately struck by how hard it was to join what was going on as I had no knowledge of previous issues. This was a situation that would be repeated regularly as people came and went. It was like being an outsider looking through a window into an intense room yet still able to hear what was being said. There was also extreme consternation among those present about the young woman who had been brought in for the weekend. She was due to go that evening.

As she went and the others returned, that sentiment seemed to move up a gear into almost open rebellion. Galvanised by a physically imposing, strong willed and heavily accented woman whom I'd not met before, there was now an open split between staff and patients. It seemed that this decision had been made by the charming, intelligent, witty yet mysterious man whom I'd yet to meet again since my arrival. It became clear that day that his word went with no argument; he had absolute power over that place. Over the coming weeks I would hear him called many things. Very quickly I simply began to refer to him as god.

My sleeping problems had always revolved around an inability to get to sleep. The only real exception to that was the time I spent with Becky just after leaving the Palace when I could neither get to sleep nor stay asleep. It had taken ages to stop the infernal call of "it's 8 o'clock, time to get up" and when left to sleep I stayed asleep. Being there meant being up, ready, and able to concentrate by 9.30 in the morning. That weekend there had been no need to get up but that first Monday morning was always going to be a struggle for me. I emerged very much the worse for wear after another short night's sleep early on that Monday. The first sight I saw was the girl from the weekend. I could barely make out the blade but I saw the gushing blood as she hacked at her arms in an uncontrollable rage. I'd known cutters before, mainly those who cut because their voices told them to, but had never actually seen it happen. It was usually such a private thing. I would meet many more there and realise over time that their motivation was markedly different to that of those I'd known before. That was my baptism of fire at the ward.

As the week unfolded, the pattern and routine of the place emerged. Each morning we all met for an hour. Within that context there was variation. Two mornings a week it was us and whichever members of staff were on duty; once we split into two smaller groups; once we met alone; and once we had the community group where all staff who wanted to come could come. That was very intimidating. I hated the larger groups and rarely spoke in that context; we were at our freest when on our own. One of the aspects I found most difficult to deal with was constantly being watched and reported on. I wasn't really consciously aware of them writing things down but they were doing it. I'd learned long before in my academic career that it really is impossible to be objective. All actions are interpreted by others and therefore tainted. However much we try to be objective, the act of writing things down is by its very nature subjective. Writing things down is about judgement. That was what they were doing and I'd always hated being judged even as a small child. It was even more difficult for me to deal with if I was judged to be lying. Permanent observation was only one of the pressures of that place though.

A Pillar of Impotence

On some mornings and afternoons we had other things to do. We all did Art Therapy, another baffling damnation of previous decisions. It was less structured than I was used to, and I often struggled to decide what to do. We worked for a while then talked for a while. Interesting things emerged in these sessions, and, while I quite liked doing it, I never really felt much better for it. The one session that everyone dreaded was on Thursday afternoon; that was time for Psychodrama. Doing that was damned from the start for me by the animosity displayed towards the therapist by the more dominant members of the community. I often felt sorry for the poor woman as she had had to fill the enviable and big shoes of her apparently brilliant predecessor. Most of the time it turned out to be a disaster. It only worked on two occasions during my stay, but when it did, the results were astonishing. On those two days, I would feel physically and emotionally exhausted. I also attended a relationships group one morning a week. I rather liked the woman who ran it and generally found people more willing to be open up in her presence than with others. The predominance of women there did on occasions though, make it feel like a women's group.

Despite all the group sessions the day proved to be very long. I was unaccustomed to such long days and, as time went by, that began to take a toll. I did have time to do other things though. It was not like the Palace. I was free to come and go as I pleased and that brought a sense of relief. Initially I busied myself contacting people to tell them where I was. Unsure how long I would be there, I knew how important it was for others to come and visit. Inevitably Rachel was one of the first I contacted. It was midway through my second week there that I got a message from her via the office. It was short and succinct, she was coming on Saturday. It struck me as odd that although she had the ward number, she chose to go through the staff. Immediately I was faced with my usual dilemma, I was desperate to see her but my stress levels went up. There was always fear when I heard from or faced her. That fear dominated the rest of my week.

She arrived from Cambridge late in the morning. There was a great sense of curiosity amongst those around me, who exactly was this girl who had had such a profound effect on my life? No one shared their thoughts though. We went out to sit by the Thames to drink and talk. There was nothing really out of the ordinary about this visit but she was rather inquisitive about the place and what I was doing there. A couple of hours slipped by peacefully without anything profound or alarming taking place. The eternal fear that she would stop contact did not materialise. We just had a pleasant time together. Sadly she didn't have long to stay but we parted on good terms then went back to the worlds our respective lives had dealt us: she in her home; and me in the hospital. She would be back though with very profound effects before I left London.

Gradually over the first few weeks I became more comfortable there. There were alarming moments though. I'd not been there long when the physically imposing woman who was also so dominant in the group began to probe why I was there. It was just one of those quiet evenings where there was very little to do. She was sitting with a couple of the others in the central part of the ward that doubled as a dining room.

"What's your diagnosis?" she started. Unease swept over me. It was the question I never asked.
"They say I have a Personality Disorder" was my very guarded response.
"What sort of Personality Disorder?"
I wanted to just get away; tell her to fuck off; anything to get out of the conversation. But I was just honest. "Narcissistic so they tell me."
"I'm not sure I'm going to like you." Fuck off went the thoughts, fuck off cunt. Over and over it went but I just walked away. The response of most of the others was more welcoming though. People came and went just as before but I seemed to settle in reasonably well. As at the Day Service, most of us propped each other up. And propping up was what was needed much of the time. There was always someone in a bad way, and that meant we were always all under pressure. Group Therapy had a nasty habit of opening wounds, wounds that were left open at the end of the allotted time. Together we had to fill that gap and plug the pain.

I liked to get away from it by going on long, slow, and as was my habit, simple walks. I often went along the river in one direction or another. Along to Tower Bridge and back by the Tower of London. Other times I wandered along the South Bank to where the Globe was being built. I rarely deviated from a straight path due to my fear of getting lost, but it got me away from things for a while. I also got into the habit of going to Charing Cross Road to indulge my passion for books and Chinese food. The food was always modest in value but enjoyable nonetheless. These were the few little pleasures that kept me going through the hard times.

The other great pressure that many had to deal with was meeting god himself. This was a variable but often grand affair. It could also be very intimidating. My first meeting with him was positively alarming. There was god himself, his junior Doctors whom I would quickly christen his archangels, a couple of members of the nursing staff or angels, and finally a bevy of students who seemed to worship at his feet. He did, however, maintain his original charm and seemed to be genuinely concerned. Others regularly had different stories to tell of him and a myriad of names were given to him. Few of them were polite. I seemed to see him each week, something that was noted by others and deemed to be unusual. It made no odds to me though. That would change.

It must have been about three weeks into my stay when I met someone new. One of the great irritants of my stay was having to move rooms frequently. Most of this had to do with gender and pecking order. More women were there than men so accommodation was complicated. There were two three person dormitories and five single rooms making up the capacity of eleven beds. The shortage of beds created by the Care in the Community policy seemed to have its most profound effect in London. Not only were we forced to move by new arrivals but also having beds being occupied by others at weekends when many of us went home meant that valuables had to be packed up each time. What everyone wanted was a single room, and that depended on how long one's stay had been. I'd been lucky and unlucky on my arrival, I was put in a single room but it was close to the main road and as such was extremely noisy; that, of course, exacerbated my insomnia. I was moved fairly quickly to what was usually a male dormitory. That too would change as the balance of the genders shifted over time. It was during my first stay there that I met the new arrival. I walked in one afternoon to find an unknown woman lying face down on the bed next to mine on the other side of the partition. She sobbed quietly. I had no idea who she was but clearly she was very unwell, and even more distressed. Without looking up she asked me to talk to her. Slowly she stopped crying and turned to face me. Her long blonde hair framed a beautiful face. She was young yet older than me. I put on *All About Eve* very softly on my stereo and she seemed to respond further to that, calm coming slowly over her. Distress slipped away as the tape rolled on.

"This is a beautiful song" I said as it progressed.

"Not as beautiful as when I sing it." And with that she very quietly sang. It was more than beautiful. That is how I met the singer. She was from the ward downstairs. Over the coming weeks she became a constant friend, one who was not tainted by the pressure we felt day by day, living on that ward. It was with her that I first entered the pub that separated us from the deafeningly busy main road beyond the courtyard that caught the sun late in the morning as spring moved towards summer. The pub was a gay pub, and it would, in time, become a regular haunt for the men and women of the ward, regardless of their sexuality.

I learned within but a few days that issues of sexuality were a major theme underpinning much of the work that was done in the place. I would see many people go in with one sexual orientation and leave with another. Others were aware of their orientation but struggling to come to terms with their lives and relationships. It was, in a sense, strange to be one of the few males in a predominantly female world. This would later lead to difficult sexual undertones going around, particularly towards the end of my stay. I'd mainly stayed well clear of women since Rachel. This was something one of the archangels brought up once. Why hadn't I found another girlfriend? This was an idea I wrestled with from time to time. But there were two major stumbling blocks to that. Firstly I was acutely aware of the effect she would have on such a relationship. I didn't want to impose what went on in my head on anyone else. The second and perhaps more significant block was the rather odd and deeply unpleasant experience of her voice in my head going crazy. On the rare occasions that I had become involved with other women since then the voice changed what it had to say. Most of the time she said the same things over and over in random order. When there were other women around her voice became much more threatening and aggressive and deviated from its normal path. And that was an awful experience that would repeat itself for the duration of my madness.

The other rather darker but related theme was sexual abuse. There were many there who had suffered at the hands of such people, often by their own family members. It was not anything new to me as I had been very close to such a victim a few years before. Yet it was the most moving and often harrowing aspect of the ward that we had to deal with. There was usually a great deal of support but at times the biting arena of the group took its toll. So often the stories were accompanied by extreme self harm, be it from the blade of a knife or razor, or in other cases by the bottle. Whether it was drink, drugs or blade, it seemed to be the only way of attaining relief from their pain for so many. Abuse was a word that sat very uneasily with me, whatever form it took.

My period of relative stability stayed with me for the first few weeks in London. To an extent this was a bad thing to happen as they were unable to see what things were like at their worst for me. How much of it came out when I talked in the smaller groups was difficult to gauge. But the darkness was still underlying my existence, it just didn't show in an obvious way. It was under these circumstances that my next clash with the powers that be occurred. God wasn't there that day and I was seeing the more junior of his archangels in his stead. Since that very first weekend when they had raised the idea of increasing the medication, nothing more had been said. Wondering what was going to happen I decided to raise it.

"Are you going to increase my medication?" I enquired rather nonchalantly.
"We don't want you to become too dependent on medication" came the rapid and rather hostile response. Stunned by the comment I followed up the enquiry.
"It doesn't make a difference to me whether you change it or not, I was just wondering why you hadn't done what you said you would do."
"I'll increase it to two pills for three weeks but I don't think it will make any difference."

I was still blissfully unaware of the game that god was playing, and his belief that I didn't have an illness, merely a disordered personality. This was the first time that I saw the archangels in action, controlled by god and often acting simply as his mouthpiece. Angered though I was I just let it drop. I really didn't give a shit about the increase but I did care about the accusatory way in which the exchange had been handled, and I was not impressed that they seemed to be underestimating just how painful my existence was. The pills would again come back to haunt me later and another crack in my relationship with god's people would appear.

The stability period ended abruptly after about a month. The slump was rapid and devastating. There was no warning and no explanation as to why. That, of course, was the first thing they asked me. All I could mumble was that maybe it was being stuck there as an in patient. Maybe the pressure had got to me, maybe it was the tiredness caused by the work or the early mornings. They remained unconvinced and in retrospect, it is highly likely that they thought I was faking it and manipulating them. That was far from the truth. The reality for me was that yet again I was in mental freefall. As ever when this happened I became more and more withdrawn from things going on around me. I became entirely introverted and communicated less than usual. Physically the effects were equally dramatic. The head and eye pain became more extreme. The exhaustion increased and I was back in the cycle. Sleep became harder to achieve and with that my condition worsened.

The other patients seemed very concerned and rallied round. There were always offers of help but little they could do. They did care though. The singer was always there for me. I remember physically removing myself from an Art Therapy group and sitting by the door. The session just washed over me but at the end one of the others came over and all she said was "I just want to give you a hug." That seemed very odd to me but she went ahead all the same. The response from the team was limited or non existent. God didn't seem to be at all concerned and they were mainly standing off from the situation. They just didn't seem to get it, but then there always was a gulf between them and us in any such facility; they were still the enemy.

May started slowly and painfully. The early mornings seemed merely to prolong the agony. Nothing was shifting just the constant throb in the head, the suicidal urges and her voice. Minutes seemed to take hours as I looked on remotely to reality. Day after day, it was all the same. Patients came and went as ever and others were suffering too. In particular one of the day patients came in for a while. He was very intelligent and interesting to talk to. He also had very severe manic depression. Like me he was a Cambridge man, but in contrast, he'd hated it, got ill and left. Older than me, two different ages and paths crossed when I'd met him, different routes to the same place. We suffered together.

It was pouring with rain that Saturday morning in May. It was FA Cup final day, Chelsea against the all conquering Manchester United on their way to the double. Some had gone home for the weekend. I had not. I'd never really been interested in gambling but we were all talking about the game and decided to place some small bets on the result. There was a bookies just out on the main road and the two men of Cambridge went naively in. Bewildering was what came to mind, it seemed impossible to merely place a bet backing one team or the other but we had to name the score as well. Surprised we just scribbled down some made up scores, paid our money and left.

It was a terrible day for me, my mind was racing and my head pounding. I had become almost oblivious to the pain as it was there all the time, but that day it was excruciating. As the hours ticked away to kick off time the pain worsened. I never took anything for it because nothing seemed to work. The trial of the codeine had failed years before so I didn't bother with paracetamol. They were always dubious on the ward about giving out such pills. But I was desperate, anything to ease the pain. I asked, they gave, and I took. As expected it was to no avail.

The game came and went. None of us won our bets. I was still in mental and physical pain. And there was a long way to go before I could lose consciousness with the help of the blue and white capsules. I was seized by one of my frequent yet paradoxical desires to be alone. The rain continued to pour down, but that did not deter me. They were all used to me going off alone to walk so nobody seemed concerned with me going out. I put on a light coat and took my leave of them.

In the slow monotonous gait which characterised my movements when very unwell, I crossed the road, went down the steps and headed towards the Globe. My mind raced as I went. Rachel was constantly in my head, I love the rain, I love the rain. It was just an accompaniment to the racing of my thoughts. The rain dripped off my curly hair into my eye brows and then down into my eyes. Wearing lenses and getting water in the eyes is never a good idea so I had to constantly wipe it away. Slowly onward I moved, barely aware that the path was deserted. Who after all would go out in weather like that unless it is important? This was important though. I had to get away but I could never get away from myself. I just wanted the pain to stop. I didn't really know where I was going, merely that I was heading in the direction of the Globe.

I stopped short, walked to the edge of the low parapet and stared out over the water. What would it be like to drown? Would it be quick? Would the impact stun me if I jumped from a bridge? On I stared and my thoughts washed over me. I love the rain, I love the rain. Those words over and over, in that soft yet echoing voice. The rain was soaking through my clothing. Could I jump? Should I jump? Do I want to jump? I want to die. Why won't it stop? I love the rain. Can I do this?

It came out of nowhere. It was quiet at first but grew louder as the minutes slipped by. Time to die it said, time to die. It was different. It was a new voice, the deep voice of a man. I didn't recognise it. Time to die. It vied with her voice for dominance, but it could not put her down. They never spoke in unison, they just settled into a rhythmic, terrible duet. Time to die. I love the rain. Time to die. I love the rain. His voice was louder and more menacing. Still they went on, on and on. My head pounded and my thoughts went on. Who is this man? You want to die. Can I do it? I want to die. The voice urged me on but I just stood there. I don't know if anyone was around, I was lost in my own world. Neither do I know what stopped me from jumping. How long I was there for is also a mystery.

I wandered slowly back to the ward with the voices still going. A young man of twenty four, soaked to the skin who'd been so close to death just a few minutes before. I had to change when I got back. There was a new voice abroad, one that I didn't understand. But he was my voice and they were never going to know of him. That voice would plague me only when I was at my worst, and it came back for the next seven years.

A Pillar of Impotence

It was May 1994. Manchester United had just won the FA Cup. The slaughter was well underway in a place in Africa that few of us knew about; within a few short weeks nearly a million people would be dead. The man called Fred and his alleged deeds were still all over the papers. People were still fascinated by those events. He was in jail, never to be convicted; his wife would be in due course. And I was back in the place I had come to call the Hotel California. I was always free to come and go, just as I had done that late afternoon in May, but I could never really leave. How could I give up what was realistically the last medical option to stop the pain? The pain went on as did the rain.

Chapter 18

Into the Bearpit

It was on one of my early meanderings along the South Bank of the Thames that I came across it. On a rare, and for me, daring detours from the direct route I found a building with a plaque attached to its wall. From what little I knew of London or more particularly Elizabethan London, I was aware that the South Bank had been a play ground to the people. Taverns, brothels, and play houses had dotted the area, and the reconstruction of the Globe, all be it in the wrong place, was the prime evidence of this place's past. Here, on the wall of what looked like a very insignificant building, was another and much less ostentatious monument to the city's past. It marked the spot on which the Elizabethan Bearpit had stood. It struck a chord with me immediately, although I wasn't initially able to pinpoint why. As time continued during my stay at the ward, a clarity emerged. Sitting day after day in the group in the mornings and so often seeing wounded souls torn further to pieces by the others, the noble beast of the pit came to mind; desperately fighting an uneven contest, chained physically as it was taken apart by the dogs. It seemed a strangely apt description of the ward. We weren't chained physically, but we were all aware that it was the last chance. Yet there was this apparent philosophy that they had to break what was left in us. The breakers could the staff, the patients, or indeed both; our own dogs. And at the helm was god. I lived in fear of being cast into the pit, but subconsciously knew already that one day I probably would be.

In the six or so weeks after the new voice arrived in my head, critical shifts would occur in my relationship with those around me, and ultimately my fate at the ward would be decided. My weekly meetings with god or his archangels continued but they began to change rapidly. He became predictably unpredictable. I saw for the first time the charm disappear and the anger that others had told me of begin to emerge. It appeared to go into a pattern, one week the charm, the next aggressive challenges. But even that wasn't always the case and I learned to never know exactly what to expect from him. The aggressive meetings were truly frightening. He seemed intent on making me angry and breaking me down. I would never let that happen. In his mind I was playing games with him and he once directly put that to me. That was very far from the truth, I was merely telling my story in the same way that I had always done, and tried to do the best I could to express how I felt at the time. He was playing the games not me.

As this drama played itself out over the next few weeks, life at the ward continued as normal; and there normal could be very disturbing. I did, however, have a number of visitors. The Cambridge guys came, as did old school friends. Steve took me to see *Schindler's List* and then on to the famous Wong Kei. Moving as it was, I found it disturbing and vowed that I would not see it again; I was wrong on that one. Musical friends came alone and in groups. Tom came over from Kent and we sat in glorious sunshine in the court yard of an ancient pub passing the time over beer. Then there was the memorable visit of Chris from Cambridge in which lunch took three hours and involved huge quantities of Thai food. More importantly it allowed me to miss a particularly disastrous afternoon of Psychodrama. I returned to find the ward deserted and that all of them had adjourned to the neighbouring pub to get over the experience. My parents came once, and Miriam a couple of times. It was these visits, and my travels that helped me to stave off the pressure.

That pressure continued as did my instability. As well as me there were others in crisis and we had to try to keep ourselves together. Day patients came and went as beds became vacant. It was during one in patient stay that I did learn something very significant. As happened so often the relationships group was dominated by the issue of abuse. I sat there one morning listening to a particularly harrowing story from a woman who had been brought in for a while. Older than me, I'd always liked and got on well with her. Here she was telling her story in words rather than her weekly variants in the art therapy session on the same theme.

"Did your mum know?" asked one of the company.
"She did but she thought it only happened once or twice."
"Once is once too often." It just came out of me without even thinking about what I had said. Then I realised just how significant that comment was. Once was once too often. I had always been acutely aware of my past and I always felt that that insight

sometimes hindered the potential of talking therapies. After all, how could I change the past? I had heard many stories of abuse in many forms but the idea had been one that I struggled with. I knew even at the time that there is something very wrong about repeatedly hitting nine year old children about the face and head. It was the price, and a very secret one we paid for being part of a world famous choir. It wasn't an every day occurrence, but living with the shadow of that was, for us, the norm. Yet my experiences had always paled into insignificance in comparison to much that I had heard in the past three years. Yet that one little, off the cuff sentence changed that perception. Abuse was abuse, and it was the effect it had on the recipient that was significant. It was, perhaps, the one really significant concept that I learned in London. A small breakthrough.

As summer came there were lighter moments. The singer was a continued source of fun and laughter. The trips in the evening to our more rowdy neighbour became an almost nightly if brief custom. It was always a strange feeling being desired by those that I didn't desire, but that seemed to be the norm in what little I knew of the gay world. I was almost always accompanied by others, predominantly women. This elicited the interesting complaint put to me there one night that I was "taking too many women" there. It was a wholly more alarming experience going there alone. On one of those rare occasions I received as volley of invites all of which I had to decline on the grounds, legitimate ones of course, that I had to get back for my medication. The little blue and white capsules now served another purpose. And then there were the medical exams.

I suppose it must have been early in June when we were asked if any of us would like to be patients for the medical student's practical Finals. We would of course be paid a small appearance fee, and given the precarious nature of surviving on benefits which could be cut after a lengthy stay in hospital, it seemed an interesting proposition. I also thought it might be quite fun and lift the continuing gloom for a couple of hours at least. All I knew was that the students would be given a chance to meet and talk to a patient with one of three types of illness, one of which was psychiatric. They would then go and talk to the examiners, and if necessary, the patient could be called in as well. Having agreed to take part, I was given instructions merely to turn up at a different part of the hospital at a certain time.

Having just about made it there I sat down next to two well dressed young men. We exchanged greetings and pleasantries and then they carried on their conversation. It seemed obvious to me that they just thought I was another student. The thought that I might be one of the patients didn't seem to have entered their heads.

"God I hope I don't get a psyche patient" one said. "I really don't know much about that."
"I know what you mean, neither do I." A wicked internal smile swept across me. It appealed to what was left of my sense of humour that I had deceived them. Having said that, on nearly all stays or visits to the nuthouse, I had been mistaken for a Doctor. There would be more of that later in the summer.

The two men were called away to their respective rooms. Wishing them both luck I just sat there. A few minutes later the organiser called me and directed me into a room. There he was, the student who'd made the comment. There was a look of horror on his face. My smile grew broader.

"How did you present?" was his opening line. Odd thing to say I thought, but then we started. As the story unfolded he overcame his obvious discomfort and gave a very good account of himself.

Over the next couple of days I had a number of such interviews and their quality was variable. There were some very interesting and memorable meetings though. There was the woman who was so nervous she could barely speak. I spent the next three quarters of an hour slowly and methodically taking her through what she needed to know. The knowledge was all there, she was just overcome by fear.

Then there was the young Asian woman who was quite brilliant but bemused by the end. She was to come out with two memorable comments that would always stick with me.

"You're a nice patient, at least you can speak" she commented part the way through the examination. We talked some of the diagnosis of Personality Disorder and she seemed initially to take it all in.

As we moved towards the end of our meeting she was given her five minute warning. We carried on. Then her alarm came forth.

"I'm not sure I understand this thing about a Personality Disorder."
"Neither do I but I'll tell you what I know." There then followed a frantic and confused potted history of my limited knowledge. Still looking concerned she was called away. I didn't have to go to see the examiners so I assume she must have done okay. On the way out I commented to the organiser, a psychiatrist herself, and a nicer one than most, what I had said at the end.

"Oh God, you didn't mention that did you?" With that we both smiled.

It was, on the whole, a memorable, intriguing and enjoyable couple of days. I certainly never regretted the experience. I would subsequently agree to be filmed for training purposes. Motivated again by dwindling and uncertain resources I agreed to take part. That was a decision I would bitterly regret. For years after I would be plagued by two separate yet intertwined visions, one that it would be seen by someone I knew, and the other that it would be shown in a lecture and that the lecturer would tell the students that I was a liar. Fear of such judgement continued to haunt me long after I had left the Hotel California behind.

June also brought a most unexpected turn of events. It would be a critical turning point in my time in London. I'd always liked Pat who had key worked me since my arrival. She had been caring and compassionate from the start and shared my passion for Bob Marley and regularly danced in that inimitable West Indian style when I played it in the day room. It was in the early part of June that she surprised me by calling me into one of the private rooms as she needed to ask me something.

"Rachel has been on the phone and she wants to talk to the Doctors. We need your consent for that to happen." How curious. They might start to believe me. That must be a good thing. The thoughts came rapidly to me. It can only do some good. None of the thoughts were against the idea, indeed, all of them seemed to support the notion.

"I've got no problem with that." It was just a matter of waiting then but I realised it would not be long as she was reaching the critical exam time within the next week or two.

The following Monday god was back to his old charming self. There was the usual bevy of hangers on in the room. He asked if it would be okay to talk to her as they needed my permission. Again I replied that that would be fine, adding that they were quite free to tell her things I'd said to them. He assured me that they would never do that as such things were confidential. That struck me as odd as I was quite willing for it to happen but I let it pass. Things were still very bad for me both mentally and physically but the idea provided a tiny glimmer of hope as I left his court.

Later that same week I lay on my bed alone in the dormitory. It was the afternoon. I was consumed with my thoughts and the fighting of the two voices, totally shut down from all around me. There was quiet knock at the door that took a while for me to register.

"Mark," said a quiet almost inaudible voice. "Mark, it's Rachel." I heard her voice so much of the time yet I was unable to recognise it in the real world as it was so unexpected. No one had warned me that she was coming that day. She'd just made the arrangements and come down to talk to them without my knowledge. There she was in the room and real. Almost instantly the voices stopped and I was alive again, with a genuine physical form before me. I was just pleased to see her. She explained that she didn't have a lot of time but she would like to go out for a drink.

I think we went back to sit by the river for an hour or so and just talked quietly. There were no revelations really. She explained that she had spoken to both god and one of the archangels and had been very impressed with them. She didn't reveal what they had talked about but seemed pleased with the outcome and that it had been a worthwhile effort. As her time was precious the meeting was all too short. But it was friendly and I left her at the station feeling a little better for having seen her. Then it was back to what passed for reality in my world. I was as yet unaware of how significant the conversation between the three of them would be in sealing my fate there. That would have to wait until the next couple of meetings with god and his minions. Only then would the extent of immense damage that had been done that day in early to mid June emerge.

Mid June also brought with it the start of the fourth year since the birth of my madness. Much had happened since that long ago day, a day that had started with joy, expectation and guilt. The events of the last day of the Bumps played so often in my mind. In four years I'd never found any way to control the flashbacks or that haunting voice. She'd been there for real and I'd not recognised her. The pain had grown more intense over those many months but no solution seemed to appear. Nothing had shifted in my time at the Hotel, I'd just seen people come and go and no one seemed to make much progress. In fact, I had regressed into one of the most intense periods of distress I'd ever suffered. How I'd survived that wet day on the Thames eluded me, and much of me wished that I hadn't. At least I'd seen Rachel.

The magnitude of my error in letting her come to talk to them was revealed the following Monday morning. He was smiling as I went in. Around was a smaller group of worshipers than usual; as ever they sat there listening to the every word of the master. He spoke of how delighted he was to have finally met Rachel. Then he gave his conclusion. He didn't reveal exactly what was said to him and his archangels but the gist was that she couldn't possibly have had a relationship with me as I wasn't a Christian. Moreover this fitted precisely with his theory of what had happened. It was all, apparently, my delusion, I'd simply fallen in love with the wrong person. Game, set, and crucially, match to god. Now all that was necessary was to work on getting over it. The great one had spoken.

I was stunned and instantly realised I'd made a terrible mistake. It was just so at odds with how things seemed at the time. Maybe I was deluded, but then again, it would have had to have been a mass joint delusion shared by many people. I struggled on during the meeting but to no avail; that was that.

That I was not completely deluded was confirmed a few days later when Becky came to visit. She had been a fairly regular visitor since my arrival in March as she now lived close by. Crucially at the time she had been living with Rachel and they were good friends. When I told what I had been relayed to me by god, her response was swift and emphatic.

"Bullshit. She was completely obsessed with you." In god's eyes Becky must have been deluded as well. There were others too who would have confirmed it. But then again, with the exception of Rachel, no one ever bothered to talk to anyone who had known me before I became ill. I would learn later that when I had been taken to the Palace nearly three years before, Miriam had been there and they had point blank refused to talk to her. She was the one person there who really knew anything about me, yet she was of no interest to anyone. Shortly after the fateful meeting between god and Rachel, he would speak to Miriam, but not only would he dismiss her, he would blatantly lie to her. Chris would also offer to talk to him but nothing would come of that either. But that was in the future and I was still struggling with both the present and the past.

The war in the Bearpit continued apace. There seemed to be what for us was an alarming trend of ever younger people being sent there that summer. Fifteen was apparently the age of consent there, a trend that did not go unnoticed in the therapy groups. The Bearpit was a very frightening place to be at times and we were all concerned that patients so young were being exposed to it. But then it wasn't really up to us; he spoke, they all obeyed. I in turn kept my usual dignified silence in the large groups. But my time was coming.

Outside of group though, most of us were great friends. In my hour of need I continued to enjoy great support from everyone. Others too relied on the solace and compassion of those of us who shared our own terrible experiences. The trips to the pub had become brief but nightly events now. We never stayed long or drank much but it was just our way to unwind from the constant pressure of the place. Pressure often told but there was always a welcoming arm after battle. The singer still always there for me and others, and much to our collective relief, she was getting better. The sun also brought a sense of some joy and we were often to be found along the banks of that great river just sunning ourselves and surprising passers-by. But the help and support was not easily accepted some of the time. We climbed the hospital tower one day to look at the magnificent vista of that huge city. Whilst there, I was seized by an incredible desire to be completely alone. Yet I could never be alone there. I'd often desired to be alone but this far more intense than anything I'd ever felt before. To the obvious concern of those with me I simply fled. After a couple of hours the feeling simply died slowly away. That was a uniquely terrifying moment that fortunately was never to be repeated.

We were well into summer with the approach of July when they made their pivotal move. I'd just started what god called Cognitive Analytical Therapy with one of the nurses. In retrospect this was designed to rid me of my apparent delusion. I still saw Pat on a one to one basis, but had also started being dual worked by one of the others. Younger than Pat, she was an interesting and clever woman and I rather enjoyed talking to her. It was at one of our meetings that their plan was unveiled.

"We were wondering if you would think about considering moving to one of the ward houses. It's your choice and just something to think about that will make things easier on the funding front." That's not a choice it's an ultimatum. It's an ultimatum. It's an ultimatum. Over and over the thought came. There is no choice. It's been decided. The thoughts continued long after we had finished. And they were alarming thoughts.

That night I spoke to both my parents and Miriam and conveyed exactly what I thought. In subsequent days they all spoke to god without my knowledge and out of their own convictions. All three were reassured that it was my choice. The lie was exposed at the next ward round.

I walked in to find god smiling and happy. That was in sharp contrast to some of the recent my experiences. Still smiling, he opened simply.

"So when are you moving to my house then?"
"I'm not sure that I am."
"But what choice do you have?" I was right, I was right. It was indeed an ultimatum. Then darker thoughts swept over me. He lied. He lied. He lied to them. He lied to Miriam. The effect was devastating. Rage engulfed me. But I knew I was trapped. I did what I was told or all hope was lost. There would be no more treatment

after this. And that was as big a dilemma as whether to live or die. Rachel's intervention had come to fruition. At the same time, an irretrievable crack had opened in the relationship, one that amplified all the smaller ones that had developed over the previous three months. He had lied directly to those I cared about. Yet the dilemma still remained. I left deep in thought.

That day marked the beginning of the end at the ward. Gradually increasing and constant pressure was put on me by the whole team. They did it in different ways but it was always there. And controlling it all was god. My relationship with him turned into almost open warfare. He told me that he didn't think I would ever find a medication that would help. He then asked me if I was taking my medication at weekends. He said it with a friendly smile, a question brought about by their insistence that I bring none with me leaving a month's supply back in Kent; it was hard to use that amount when I was only there for a few weekends. It seemed an utter contradiction on his part; if they weren't helping why be concerned about me not taking them. The fact that I struggled so much to sleep without them did not seem to have had a bearing on their thinking. All the time he seemed to be trying to provoke me into revealing my anger. That was a pleasure I was not prepared to let him have.

The idea of moving there was an alarming one. The house itself was around half an hour away on the bus. London was place that still scared me; I was even more alone there than I had been in Kent. The house was shared with others from the ward and from another hospital. There was no direct support there at all. As a result, there was little that could be done in a crisis to help. Their response to that concern was a simple one, "you can always phone the ward." That, I knew would not be enough. It was back to the age old dilemma of mental health in general: it's only acceptable to have a crisis in office hours. That was a complaint I would come across hundreds of times in my many years in the System. Above all of that though was the thought that I couldn't see where this treatment was going. There had been so many let downs in my eyes that I couldn't see how we could paper over the considerable cracks that had emerged. I struggled to trust people anyway, but there was now a deep feeling of mistrust when it came to them. On the other hand, I was acutely aware that what lay in wait for me back in Kent was something akin to oblivion. If the best treatment available had failed for whatever reason, there was little hope left. As the pressure increased so did that mistrust.

There was something else troubling me that June which presented an equally difficult dilemma. Lisa was an old school friend of mine who hailed from Cayman. Educated in England she had returned to Cayman to work shortly after graduating from university. The result of which was that I hadn't seen her for a few years. That summer she was back in England for a while and I received an invitation to a party at the house of her future husband in Surrey. I was torn in my usual way when it came to decisions, I desperately wanted to catch up with her but I feared the questions that would inevitably come up. A favourite in the past from people from the Cambridge background had been "so where are you based?" The moment I was asked such a question or was asked what I did I always froze. It was the nightmare scenario of so many with a mental illness, a disability that was very real but could not be seen. There was always the implication in my mind that I had to justify my existence, prove my value to society. I knew there would be Cambridge people there along with many others from very similar backgrounds. Somehow, if I went, I would have to fend such things off, and that would almost certainly mean lying. I suppose no one was really interested in the response but they were enquiries that played havoc with my mind. What would I do? What would I say? Pressure. Distress. Fear. That was what I would feel.

But it wasn't just that I wanted see them, it that I felt I had to see them. That made it even more complicated. I talked a great deal to the others about how I felt and feared. One offered to come with me but I thought she wouldn't quite know what to make of such people. They even asked if I wanted to do a Psychodrama about it but it seemed far too self centred an issue to use that time for, just too small and irrelevant to do. Perhaps I was wrong on both counts but in the end I did go, and go alone. It proved to be relatively relaxing to start with. Then the test came.

"What do you do then?" came the question from one of two Scotsmen whom I'd stumbled across. I just decided to be honest, brutally honest.

"I'm on weekend release from a psychiatric unit in London." They looked shocked for a moment, then responded.

"No you're not, you're a Doctor aren't you?"

"No, honestly, I'm on weekend release from hospital." They didn't believe me. On it went for nearly an hour. At that point Lisa passed by on her travels.

"Is this true?" said one of them.

"Oh yes, it's true." With that they just seemed to accept it and carry on with their drinking and conversation. I rather enjoyed that exchange, a very rare treat for me.

Acceptance was not always straightforward. There was another occasion when chance threw me into such a conversation. It was equally farcical but with rather more unpleasant undertones. The entrance to the little courtyard that caught the sun was flanked on one side by the pub and on other by a newsagent's. Between the newsagents and the road was public phone box. In an age when the mobile phone was both rare and bulky not to mention very expensive, mere mortals such as myself were reduced to using such boxes if all else failed. We had a pay phone on the ward but that June it had broken down. So it was that I found myself one hot and sunny afternoon heading through the archway, turning to my right and walking towards the aforementioned box. It was but a minor irritation to find it occupied. I just stood and waited. I was startled to feel someone walk straight into me. Turning apologetically I was confronted with a very familiar face. Before me stood a Kuwaiti lawyer from my Cambridge days on a random London street. I'd not seen him since the day I had graduated, that fateful day three years before on which I had had my first panic attack. My mind cast back to that day as he went through the usual pleasantries we all seem to deem so necessary to our lives. I waited for the question. Sure enough it came quickly.

"What are you doing now?" Same question, same bewilderment.

"I'm in this hospital here" I said gesturing back towards the unseen unit. It just seemed to come out of me without thinking.

"Are you a Doctor then?"

"No, I'm a psychiatric patient."

"Shit, you're not going to knife me are you?" his expression having changed in an instant.

"No, of course not, why would I want to do that?" He looked increasingly nervous. Then he looked at the shop behind me.

"What are you doing here?" he said, strangely eyeing its window display.

"I'm waiting for the phone." He didn't seem to believe me.

"You're not going to do an armed robbery on that shop are you?"

"No, of course not. I'm waiting to use the phone." Still not sure we talked some more. I spoke a little of what had happened and how I'd ended up there. Then he asked a question I should have anticipated but which took me by surprise.

"Were you ill at Cambridge?"

"Yes, very."

"You did a fucking good job of hiding it." I was struck by how that comment could be construed as a good or a bad thing. On the one hand I was pleased I had done it so well. On the other, how futile had it been? The thought of seeking help earlier and how different life could have turned out occasionally occupied my mind. But when I thought about it, I always came to the conclusion that I would have had the same response that I received when I did seek help. The conclusion that I was depressed because I didn't have a job would merely have been replaced by being told I was stressed out about my finals; both conclusions, of course, would have been false.

We parted soon after but he was clearly still unconvinced by what I was doing.

"If you have any problems just let me know. I am a lawyer and I'm in that building over there." With that he headed off down the road. I simply turned to the now vacant phone box, opened the door and made my call. His nervousness was in a way understandable; it was a fear born out of ignorance. I don't suppose I would have been any different to him had it not happened to me. Many of us fear what we don't understand. I didn't understand it myself and it was certainly very frightening. But I was living it so I had to accept it.

That fear grew as the pressure grew. And that grew as we moved into July. From all sides I was pushed towards the house. The exception was the other patients. Why couldn't I cope? It was quite simple, I just moved there and came in during the day. What choice do you have? But that was just it, I couldn't cope. The refrain went on. Then things turned nasty. There was another patient who was moving to the house, one who was very vulnerable. I'd met her on my first visit. She'd been asked to show me around that first day. It was a question that clearly terrified her, but she meekly acquiesced. We got on very well in the time I was there. Then they linked my move to hers. They had reservations about her going there on her own and suggested that they would only let her move if I went as well. That was close to being the last straw. In my eyes it was totally unfair to make that link and put that kind of pressure on me. Not only unfair but utterly unprofessional. They did it anyway. I still refused to commit and she moved anyway. What I needed was wise counsel from someone who did not have a vested interest in the decision. There were only two people who I knew could give that: Heather and David. But they opposed the former. The latter was welcomed as a possible course of action if I decided to leave.

The closest I came to cracking was in ward round when god was away. I saw two of the archangels in his stead, one a Doctor and the other a senior nurse. Given their instructions they openly accused me of wasting everyone's time. I received a barrage of criticism throughout. The rage was at its height but I refused to let them see it. I merely held out and thanked them for their time after, as was my custom. I think that really pissed them off. When I spoke to the others after about what had happened they were stunned. But the archangels were playing god's game and losing. Despite his angry outburst of "stop playing games with me" that he had levelled at me in one meeting, I was never anything but honest with them. Perhaps it was all my delusion. All the while god refused to give me a diagnosis on the grounds that "you might think you can find a better shrink who might be able to help you."

Behind the scenes in the brevity of the weekends in Kent I was able to make an arrangement to see David at Barming. He couldn't see me until the Monday morning. Ordinarily, if any us went home for the weekend, we were due back on the Sunday evening as Monday morning group was sacrosanct. Due to the exceptional circumstances I called the office to explain the situation. Pat answered the phone and said that that was fine. I would come back on Monday afternoon after my meeting. My last comment on the phone was to ask her to tell everyone I'd be back then. This she agreed to do.

I met with David that Monday morning. As ever, he was cordial and helpful, and was quite willing to take me back on if I chose to leave the Hotel. Pleased that I had some sort of option, I journeyed back on the train feeling that at least someone was there to help and support me. I entered the ward late in the afternoon and was quite shocked by the reception I got. A close friend immediately berated me for not telling her what my plans were and wanting to know why another female patient had known before her. All I'd done was talk to a member of staff and asked her to pass a message on to the patients. The weird sexual vibe caused by being the only male in an all female environment had struck. There had been dalliances in my time there but I was never sure what to make of them. There was another male there at the time but he was desperately ill and unable to communicate. Nine women and me. God knows what would have happened if I'd called the patients' phone. This was very unfamiliar territory.

And still I hadn't had the chance to speak to Heather, the one person I knew of who would able to look at my predicament with even a modicum of objectivity. I had not intended to go back to Kent the following weekend. I had a CAT session booked on the Friday afternoon. I had made no arrangements to collect medication, my own supplies having run out. But something came up that necessitated a short notice return. I don't recall what it was but it may have been an opportunity to talk to Heather. It was the middle of July. I went to bed on the Thursday night thinking that I would have to tell the CAT man that I couldn't make it that afternoon, and to ask them for some pills for the weekend. I woke up on the Friday morning and headed for the group. It was 9.30 a.m. on a Friday in July. I was completely unaware that I was about to be cast into the Bearpit.

I was tired and unwell and just expected the usual long silence. Initially it was just another Friday where everyone really just wanted to get it out of the way and prepare for the weekend. That changed abruptly when very unusually one of the archangels broke the strained silence.

"You're looking pretty rough today Mark, is there anything you want to talk about?" They've set me up. It was a rhetorical question. Throughout the next hour I was subjected to a barrage of pressure designed specifically to force me to accept the move. Whatever I said was dismissed. Around the room there was silence. All but one of the others just sat there impassively. The only one who did speak added to the pressure. She was a woman I liked a great deal but she did have a habit of questioning others to deflect from her own problems. Time slowed down completely. They've set me up. That thought kept coming back to me. Run. Get out. But I wasn't going to do that. Neither was I going to show them my rage. It just went on relentlessly. Still nothing from the forum. Help me, help me. But no help came. There was no one prepared to speak out in my support. This was not sound advice, it was the advice of vested interest sent from on high. It was the Bearpit at its very worst and in middle of it I sat utterly alone.

Somehow I held out through that gruelling hour. With time up the support came flooding in. So many came to me, some with stunned looks on their faces after what they had just witnessed. But that was not the end of it as I then had to hastily arrange for my pills for the weekend and to leave a message that I wouldn't be able to make the CAT appointment. This having been done, I left. When I returned it was put to me that I had "stormed off the ward." No one believed that it was prearranged. But then again, I'm not sure they ever believed anything I said in my stay there.

I did get my impartial advice in the end. I sat down with Heather on a glorious Sunday afternoon in her back garden. In her usual way she approached things in a very calm and measured manner. We came up with a list of pros and cons to staying or leaving and she quietly wrote them down. When we had finished she put it quite simply:

"You leave." That was enough. The decision was made. I was coming back to Kent.

I met with god the following day. It was very short meeting.

"I've decided to leave."
"You can go this afternoon then if you want." It was that simple. I'd defied his will and therefore I could fuck off. The ultimatum was fulfilled, do as I say or go. I needed time though to collect my thoughts and managed to persuade him to let me stay until the end

of the week. If nothing else I needed to say my goodbyes to those who mattered most to me in the Hotel, my great friends.

We had a huge party at the pub on the last night. Then it was on to one of the patient's flats in Bermondsey to drink and smoke long into the night. I slept in an armchair that night, content and utterly wasted. They partied on without me. There would be many more occasions such as this in that flat in the years to come; the connections were that great.

The following morning, weighed down with the accumulation of things collected over a four month stay in London, I headed for the station. It was the 30th July 1994. Treatment was over. The world had finally done something to stop the killings in Africa. Nothing much had been done to stop it in Europe though. A couple of months before, the country had been stunned by the premature death of a political figure. An obscure new man was rising in politics and along with him, a new concept. His name was Tony Blair; the concept was called New Labour. Man and concept would, in time, change our lives. As I sat on the train, facing a very uncertain and bleak future it mattered not. I was still stoned.

Chapter 19

Two Spliffs A Day Keeps Insanity Away

Cannabis Sativa is a plant with many names, many uses, and many extraordinary properties. It has been known for centuries, both as a wild plant, and as one that has been cultivated by various societies for a number of different uses. Those properties have been both revered and feared, its value or danger being very much in the eye of the beholder. In my society, at least from the perspective of those with power, it is widely feared; as a result it has been banned for some of its uses all of my life. That, however, has not stopped it being smoked by many.

I'd never come across it at school, nor indeed, any other substance with unusual properties. Unlike the post school worlds of many of my friends, in my little part of the slightly bigger world that is Cambridge, it was not something I came across very often. No one I knew had it regularly and people were rather apathetic towards it. I saw more of it in the travels of my madness but again not very often. I'd never really been much of a smoker but it did have one very extraordinary effect on me; it stopped my symptoms. In fact voices and suicidal thoughts and urges seemed positively absurd when I smoked. The pain just left me.

I was determined to do two things when I left the Hotel, buy some hash and read my medical notes. To me the former seemed the only way to survive. The latter was to get an explanation, to try to make some sort of sense of the last three years that had been the treatment phase.

Life looked very bleak after discharge. There was no obvious way forward, just waiting for the inevitable day when the voice would get too loud and the pain too great and then the pills. It was hard to look beyond the pain of now, and all the help that was available had been exhausted. Perhaps foolishly, I never took David up on his offers of help. I just couldn't see any path to follow. Often I thought of calling the Samaritans, but that was out as I didn't have free access to the phone; there was always someone around and my life was still my secret. As the evenings progressed, it was time to take refuge, down to the little quiet club, one spliff on the way and one on the way back. I never drank much, just two drinks, then back. That staved off the pain for another day. Then I had to wake up again.

I had a new shrink now. She was short and often hostile. It was she who had kept James in the Palace for so long. She had nothing to add, just trying to hinder. It was abundantly clear that her attitude was that there was nothing that could be done, and that god was right. I wasn't ill I had a disordered personality. I was just a fuck up who was beyond redemption. I never met anyone at the time who had any faith, trust or affection for her. There was no one I met who felt she had ever helped, or indeed, cared for them. Many years later I did meet one but he was the lone exception. We called her the Evil Pixie. To most of us she seemed positively evil.

I went back to the Day Service but in a very much restricted manner; little was made accessible to me. I saw Tom about once a month and that was okay but we never made any progress. He cared but couldn't see a way forward either. I did value him for the former. Always friendly and engaging it did nevertheless seem an exercise in futility. Futility or not it was essential to me that someone cared and someone tried. And that he did.

Spending less time there though presented other problems. I was able to return to getting up when I woke up, and like many in my world, that was late. But the day was very long and sleep was hard to come by. Once I got to sleep it was better, I wasn't in pain any more. Getting to sleep though was still a problem. The blue and white capsules were a God send but they weren't always consistent. Once asleep, I slept. But what of the rest of the day? I could drink and smoke myself into oblivion, but even in my despair, I wasn't prepared to do that. They were my evening past times, and evening was a long way off from an 11 o' clock wake up. Time as well as reality was distorted by madness. Most of my days were filled up by playing computer games with James. It may not have been very productive but it passed the time and did provide some distraction from the pain. There were also others to see, others who shared our pain. And those in London provided another avenue of travel.

With the first part of my quest completed within a few days of my return, my thoughts turned to the second part. I was not certain that the notes would be made available to me but in the event, my GP was most obliging. When I enquired about seeing them he was very enthusiastic and asked me to simply make an appointment and he would ensure that a room was set aside for me.

It was late in August when I arrived at the surgery for what would prove to a most enlightening and shocking couple of hours. They handed me a great bundle of papers, pointed me in the direction of a private room and said that if I needed any assistance to just call. I shut the door and sat down. The record seemed vast even though I was only four years into my madness. Not sure where to start I simply decided to go through it all from the beginning. There was a great deal about my childhood, the time I first saw the shrinks and all the tests they ran at the age of six. Nothing too shocking there though. There were some interesting and surprisingly accurate observations on the family. Then there was a whole lot of junk to sift through.

It began to get very interesting at the time I first went into hospital. Many of the gaps that had never been explained were filled. I learned for the first time that I'd been in a coma for three days and that for some of that time I had been on a ventilator. I was struck by how resilient the body was in the face of overwhelming attack from poison. The thought was accompanied by a heavy tinge of regret, not for my actions, but by the reaction that they had caused. After all, I still wanted to die.

After that though there was a strange silence. I could find nothing at all from the Palace. Maybe it had been sent and hidden from me, maybe nothing had been done. That all seemed very mysterious. The silence ended with my arrival at the Day Service. From that point until the present, and that included the discharge papers from the Hotel, the reports defied credulity; it just described a totally different person. And some of that was bordering on the obscene. Vicky's conclusion was that I shouldn't be allowed to work with women. The error was in fact all hers; my problem with her had nothing to do with her sex, it was purely that she was absolutely appalling at her job. Her feminism shone through it all, but that had merely got in the way of her ability to do what she was paid to do.

The farce of her opinions was exposed by the fact that in London, for all its faults, I had had two female key workers, neither of whom had a problem with me.

Even more alarming though was the lengthy correspondence from the original consultant, he whom I had met but three times, and only bothered to talk to me on our third and final meeting. I came across a new expression, Psychotic Depression. I'd never heard the word psychotic attached to the word depression. I had always believed that there were major elements of psychosis in my condition but these had never been acknowledged, at least, not to me. I'd also often wondered why they hadn't tried anti psychotics on me. That was a two edged sword though, maybe they would help but I had a great fear of them having seen so many of my friends suffer the terrible side effects often associated with them. Now it seemed they had thought about it without my knowledge and rejected the idea. That would be indicative of most of my experience within the System.

But it was the last piece of paper that was most alarming. He had refused to give me a diagnosis when specifically pressed to do so. Yet there, in black and white, prior to my referral to Ashford was the diagnosis of Narcissistic Personality Disorder. It was attached to the word Borderline. I took this to mean that he was not sure. It would be some time before I was made aware that that was another closely related diagnosis. I was still oblivious as to just how damaging both diagnoses were to anyone given them. In time I would realise that they were the psychiatric get out clause, the dustbin into which the untreatable were dumped. Essentially, I was considered untreatable after the Hotel had failed. But the biggest impact on me was the exposure of his lies. He had been asked directly to give a diagnosis and he had lied. It reinforced my opinion of him. Then though, there was the paperwork from god himself.

He too had refused to give me a diagnosis on the grounds that "you might think that you could find a better shrink who could help you." At the top of one of the documents was a space for diagnosis. Filling that space in his own hand were two simple words, "Personality Disorder." Another lie in black and white. As I read further, it got worse. He wrote of our first meeting, the one in which he had keenly asked me about Cambridge entrance. The story I told him was exactly as it had been explained to me some six years before. He dismissed it as a delusion. Again and again I read that word delusion; it had come first from the shrink in Ashford and then followed repeatedly by god.

As I finished, some clarity appeared in my mind. The original consultant had had an opinion. He'd sent me to Ashford to have that opinion confirmed. I'd then been sent to London for treatment and reaffirmation of that opinion. It was cut and dried. All three had worked from a starting point and that had never been challenged. It was now gospel. Yet from reading all the information, it was clear that they were all wrong. Had anyone who really knew me read what had taken me over two hours to digest, they would have thought that this extensive archive was describing a completely different person. It simply bore no resemblance to me at all. But no one ever thought to talk to people who knew me before. The one exception of course was Rachel, and she had merely confirmed their opinions. Evidence to fit a theory, not evidence to make a theory.

I left in a state somewhere akin to shock. I simply couldn't believe what had been written. All faith in them had now been blown away. They really were the enemy now. There was no one to trust. But I was acutely aware that I was in desperate need of contact and help. I felt even more alone now. At the end of god's missive was a chilling message. He considered that there was a very significant risk of suicide in my case, it was only a matter of time. It was one I knew to be true. Life looked very bleak. Madness is often a lonely place, with death the only way out. At least he'd recognised that though. Unfortunately, even that information would be denied to me when I needed it. That would be the doing of the Pixie, but that still lay a year ahead.

At the end of August I turned twenty five. There would be no party of course, just another horrible day to get through. There was, however, something very significant about that age; the DSS paid people an extra £10 per week. It seems very little really but a 20% increase in one's income is substantial. There would be downsides to being twenty five, and those problems increased as I got older. When in one's early twenties it is often assumed that one is a student. As a student there is no real need to justify one's own existence. As my twenties waned, questions about what I did and who I was became more and more difficult to field. Comments at parties were one thing, in every day life they were another.

Turning twenty five was one means of boosting my meagre income, but just prior to my exile in London, Heather had made me aware of another way. Disability Living Allowance. No one had ever mentioned it to me before and I was blissfully unaware of either its existence or potential. I was certainly never made aware of it by any professional. In retrospect had I been given a social worker it would probably have appeared on my horizon much earlier, but since I lived with my parents, that was deemed unnecessary. Had I stayed in the capital I would have been assigned one and he or she would have helped me with the paperwork. All the others had help and received substantial sums, although all these things are relative. We'd decided to wait until the outcome of my stay before applying.

Thus it was that in August I sat down with Heather to fill in the complicated forms. There were immediate problems. There was the problem of diagnosis, Personality Disorder would net nothing and depression held little sway, the *Right Diagnosis Theory* would strike again. There was also a need to back up what I was saying with other evidence. Tom wrote a letter to support me but the shrink refused to help me. That left only my mother but that would mean showing her the paperwork and letting her into my world. And that was something I was very reluctant to do. There would be awkward questions from her but there was really very little choice. She did write but was very sceptical of what I'd written, perhaps out of fear or a refusal to accept just how bad it was for me. Getting her involved was an experience I found profoundly disturbing and one that would come back to haunt me later. With what scant support I could obtain, I sent all the papers back to Blackpool and awaited their response. As ever, I expected the worst.

Their letter arrived rather quickly, much more quickly than I'd anticipated. They would indeed award me DLA but at the lowest possible rate they could give. Whilst that was welcome and useful, the gap between the low rate and the middle rate was considerable. Almost all those I knew in my situation had been given the middle rate but not me. Certainly that was the norm for those I'd met in London. There was an appeals process which I chose to exercise. It would though take time. As summer turned to autumn in 1994, I had no idea just how long it would take, nor the stress, distress, and strain that that process would exert on me.

Nothing changed that autumn. The drudgery and pain of my daily existence continued. Each night, for a few hours, it was alleviated, but in the morning, life was just as hopeless. My travels continued with my new found London friends providing an occasional time away. At these times I generally blotted out the day in a haze of drink and smoke. It seemed the only way for us to cope. I heard stories of the Hotel and sometimes plucked up the courage to go in there. I was also a frequent visitor to the pub. Everyone was pleased to see me and hopeful that I would never again have to go there. I knew I was still in need, but I was equally adamant that it would not be on their terms, and therefore I could never go back. Even after leaving we were all providing a mutual propping up service. And that autumn, we all needed each other.

I'd always been waiting for the day I lost a friend to suicide. In my world, I knew it would only be a matter of time. It was in the evening that I received the call. It was one of the girls from London, and I knew from the tone of her voice that the news was bad. It had happened, but to the least likely candidate that I could have imagined. She'd always seemed happy to me. I knew she was ill and she'd told me many stories in my time there. She was older than me and a manic depressive. Always there to support others she had seemed to be very stable in the time I'd known her. I was told that she had come in one morning very low; then she'd gone home and hanged herself. Nothing can set one up for the grief of suicide but I was remarkably philosophical about. There was so much suffering in my world, that release was just that. Peace at last. My greatest regret was that I wasn't informed in time to go to the funeral. Those still there bitterly lamented that none of them were allowed to talk about it in group. Cracks were appearing in their trust too. My first experience was painful, but it didn't stop my feelings. I also knew that it would not be the last. Sadly, there would be too many more in years to come. But then again, in my world, suicide was the norm rather than the exception.

Time ticked on. The pain went on. And my routine, such as it was, drifted on. October, November, the months when the weather is shitty but at least the daylight was reduced. With it though came the cold. It was another unexplained aspect of my condition that I was very vulnerable to extremes of temperature. I could no longer worship the sun as I had been wont to do in happier days. Nor could I tolerate any cold at all. There was nothing good on the horizon. My appeal was rejected. The next step would be to go to tribunal, and that was a prospect I feared greatly. Justify yourself. Prove that you are not a liar. The problems of a life time laid out for the sake of money. But I needed that money. What I had helped with my travel and to get through the day, but I was still very restricted in what I could do and for how long. My clothes were threadbare, shoes were an even bigger problem.

Early in December I received a most unexpected invitation. The ward was having a Christmas party and they wanted me to go. It was a wonderful chance to see old friends, but the downside was the prospect of having to see god. Having arranged to stay at the flat we'd partied at on the night of my departure, I set out with expectation and trepidation. When I had left Cambridge, it had been suggested that at some stage it would be to my advantage to return to do a Post Graduate Certificate in Education. At the time it was the last thing I wanted to do, but, over the years the idea had been reinforced by Chris. As a concept it now held some appeal but appeared to be no more than a pipedream. But it was a way of talking to god. I hated having to justify myself but now was the time to do it. In the event, god was very pleasant and rather liked the idea. There was some solidity in that path. His view on how long it would take differed drastically from mine, but the seed was sown. After that I moved off. Back to the flat and we partied on as only nutters can. The haze was everywhere. Others, of course, did the same thing, but most had far less to run away from than us. Then the morning came. Having survived the night before, I headed back to my usual oblivion. But oblivion was about to take another unexpected turn.

I went out every evening just to get away from things. Alcohol made me feel physically worse but mentally better. Smoking added to the latter effect, but not the former. But my nightly excursions were tempered by fear and paranoia. People, and more specifically their actions and questions had a very profound effect on me. They frightened me. The little club was relatively easy to deal with, particularly when stoned. Stoned brought a different paranoia, but one that was acceptable most of the time. James was much more outgoing than me though. To him, the pub at the bottom of the hill was more in tune with his needs. Occasionally he persuaded me to go there. It was there, on one such night in December that the first glimmers of reality were revealed to me.

I wondered in with my usual apprehension from the car park end. The bar was long, narrow and made from fine, old, dark wood. At the far end was an open fire, lit against the winter cold. We walked over, drinks in hand, to look for somewhere to sit. As we approached the fire, a voice greeted my companion.

"Hello James, how's it going?" The voice was confident and upbeat. Its owner had a beaming smile and striking blonde hair. Next to her, quietly in the corner sat an equally striking woman, young with long dark hair.
"Hi Laura," said James, "this is Mark." The dark girl acknowledged me then continued in her silence.
"Hi Mark, do you fancy my friend?" said Laura, "everyone else does." I wasn't sure how to react to that. I surveyed her. Troubled was the first thought. She was indeed astonishingly attractive but there was something about her. It said simply, look but don't come near. The image of a porcupine came into my head. Spikes everywhere. Here was real defence, a defence I well recognised from my past. She was untouchable.

That night was more enjoyable than most. Laura, the blonde was very outgoing and friendly. The dark Jayne was equally friendly but stood off. In time I would make my way through the quills and discover an extraordinary friend with whom I shared so much.

It was a chance meeting, one born out of fear on my part and the seeking of normality on James' part. As I headed toward what was perceived as home that night, spliff at the ready, I had little idea of what was to come. Christmas was its usual hell. New Year was little better. Occasionally as winter gave way to spring, I bumped into those two again, more occasionally I met their friends. They were splendid distractions but brief, oh too brief.

Easter was anonymous, still no tour to go on. I was going nowhere. God's prediction loomed very large most days. There was no hope.

One day I would do it. New friends or not I felt so utterly alone so much of the time. My travels were all too brief. And each night, to and from which ever drinking hole I could face on any given day, two spliffs a day kept the insanity away. Then I woke up.

As the weather warmed up and the days grew longer, I still had no idea what was about to be unleashed that summer. It has always been known since as that summer, the summer of '95.

Chapter 20

That Summer

It started merely as a trickle. As the weeks of spring drifted away and the weather warmed my forays to the bottom of the hill became for frequent. I was still very unsure much of the time and always on my guard. I still didn't stay out long or late but I gradually met a few more people. They were friends of James, and of Laura, and indeed the guarded and defensive Jayne. I was struck by their acceptance of me. I was never seen as a nutter, just another person although I had been very honest with them. There was some gratification in the normality of it all. I'd lived so long in the shadow of madness and its even more shadowy populace. We were our people but there were others out there who led what we perceived to be normal lives, the lives we'd all left behind so long ago. I was used to the dark world, painful as it was. But the world of light, of fun, and of laughter was, in some respects, even more frightening. Few of us ever felt we belonged there. It was the reality that I could see but never get to, what I strived for but was terrified of. The lengthening days of May held little portend of what was to come. By mid June I had been thrust into what the obscure political man would later call *Cool Britannia*. Joy seemed to be back in people's lives, the sombre days of recession over. For me darkness would become light for a little part of the cycle that binds us all, night follows day and day follows night.

In my previous life, mid June had been a sign of bad things to come; it meant holidays, and they were invariably awful. It also marked the death of that old life and the start of my personal plummet into hell. Every year since it started, my worst periods of illness and instability came then. In later years when I coped better some of the time, I was still very bad in mid June even when I was unaware of the date. But in 1995 it heralded not only a bout of intense pain, but also the return of the university students. I lived in what was to intents and purposes a small, quiet and insignificant town. Living such an isolated life, and never having been to school nor indeed spent much time there had left me oblivious to the extensive, intricate, almost incestuous web of inter personal connections that must exist in all such small places. From mid June

I was exposed to that for the first time. There was a youth in my town, and that summer that youth revolved around the pub at the bottom of the hill.

Despite my fears there was safety in those I knew. And with them came others they knew. From small beginnings, two girls sitting by a fire in mid winter, emerged a vast throng. They were all connected, school, friends, colleagues, brothers, sisters. The quiet, the confident. The eccentrics, the introverts. The staid, the outlandish. The hippies, the conventional. The younger, the older. More and more as the weeks passed by. Even in the middle of the week, there was always someone there. What drew us all together was fun seeking and alcohol. There was also the unwritten and unspoken side of us that was that we were running away from the troubles and boredom in our lives. It was small, sea side town hedonism.

At the weekends there was barely room to move in there, even less space to sit down. Even in the garden, on the warm evenings, having cut one's way through the haze and the tulip garden there was nowhere to sit; the floor often sufficed. But the pub at the bottom of the hill was not the only place of revelry. I'd always been struck by just how many pubs there were in such a small place. Most of them I'd never been in. There was another, totally different centre of our hedonism. Right on the beach, at the other end of town from where I resided was a bar that was equally popular. Like the labyrinth of the Palace, it had its own sentinel, the shaven headed, short but bulky karate instructor who was known universally as JB. It was his club that had brought so many of our company together. Jayne to Laura, James to both of them, and through that association of the Palace, me to all of them. Like the rest of us, JB was a night person who loved to party.

Life did not stop at closing time. There was always a house to go to, a party to attend after. Since the illness started I'd been an enforced night person also. But my nights had been so solitary, passing the time until the blue and white capsules brought a temporary end to the chaos of my mind. Now there was something to do, people to see. There was a purpose, even though it was one induced by foreign bodies. But if it stopped the pain it seemed worth it. After all, the medication I'd been taking continuously for four years was equally foreign. It had also completely failed to alleviate any of my symptoms. All it did was bring some temporary respite in the few hours when I was unconscious. No anti depressant had ever had any anti depressant effect on me. That was why I'd questioned the assumptions of the shrinks. They had too but had come up with an absurd answer, the "you're not ill you've just got a lot of problems" answer. That means you have a disordered personality. Bollocks. But they wouldn't listen.

The traditional June bout of instability was not the only problem I faced early that summer. The next stage of the battle with the DSS was about to take place. The tribunal had been set for mid July and this was the one I feared above all other. I would have sit before a panel of three people who had never met me and be judged a liar or an honest man. Judgement, that great nemesis that had plagued me since childhood. This time though, there was some help available. I'd been put in touch with a benefits expert from Social Services, and she was quite brilliant. She would handle the case for me and I just had to answer whatever questions they had for me. She was there specifically to present my case. As had been the situation with me all along, the help was not offered to me by the professionals who were supposed to do it, but by Heather's contacts. Sally set about getting the evidence together with her customary vigour, a vigour and thoroughness both feared and respected by those who sat on the panels.

It was one of the many paradoxical features of my illness that I often felt an overwhelming desire to be alone but never could be. The instability kicked in so rapidly when left for more than a few hours that I was rarely left alone. I didn't really want to live where I did but having someone around was better than having no one around. When my parents went away I always went to stay with other people, usually Miriam, although sometimes I stayed with James. If I had tried to live in a flat on my own I would probably be dead or in hospital within the space of a few days. That was precisely what the higher levels of DLA were set up to do, help for twelve or twenty four hours depending on the level of need. And it was not just me that recognised that. The comments by god that he considered me a high suicide risked backed that up. Sally duly applied to the Pixie to have the relevant document released. She refused point blank to do so on the grounds that she "wouldn't release anything I hadn't seen." But I had and she knew it. When I questioned her she told me "I can't help you." So not only was she refusing to help me she was actively hindering me. But it was what I had come to expect from them. She didn't give a shit or believe a word I said. Disordered personality again.

Even without the support of any of the professionals, Sally was confident that the case was more than solid and might even be a formality. I was not so sure. To me they were just as much a part of the enemy and it seemed in their interest not to award the money to me. They were always very secretive about how they judged things from the forms they were given. It had struck me as utterly absurd to be able to put a percentage figure on a disability as they had done to me a couple of years before. Now I was to be put on trial. As the days passed by I became more and more anxious about going. But I was just as determined to do it, to claim what was due to me. The night before I was at a party with a particularly talented and eccentric friend. That shut me off for a few hours. But the waking hours would be longer the next day as I had to get up early. That didn't help either.

It was a warm July morning when Sally picked me up for the journey once again to Ashford. They seemed quite friendly there and ushered us into a waiting room. Nervousness pervaded on my part if not on Sally's. My shakiness grew and sweat started to pour as I awaited my day in court; and that was essentially what it was. When we were called in it seemed utterly formal. There were three of them. The chairman explained the procedure and they introduced themselves, a lawyer, a doctor, and a disability worker. Sally presented the facts as they were. The doctor sat silently through the first part. Then he started. What followed was a barrage of attacks delivered with utter hostility. My mind was cast back to the hardest day in the Bearpit. On it went, the implication being that I was faking everything and I had no real thoughts of suicide. It was when he started to say "in my experience of suicide" that my mind exploded. The thoughts came as a one sided conversation. Exactly what the fuck is your experience of suicide? Do you know what it's like to contemplate the bottle? The chalkiness of the pills as they slip down your throat? Have you ever done it? Do you know what it's like to have a voice yelling "time to die" over and over? As the thought conversation went on, another part kept thinking tell it as it is. But no words would come out just short terse answers to almost unheard questions. As it had been in the Bearpit it just wouldn't stop. Much of what he said was lost in the thoughts. It just reminded me of that day as I lay helpless and unable to speak in a hospital bed being abused by a doctor in front of his students, the day of the pig. Now I could speak but I couldn't. I had to stay in control even though it harmed my case. As ever, I suffered in silence and turned my anger in on myself.

When it stopped and we were asked to leave whilst they considered their verdict I was a complete wreck. Sally looked stunned. As we went back in, I knew it was hopeless, although she kept her earlier optimism. The chairman kept it short. I'd lost by a unanimous decision. As he put it "there is no evidence." Thank you Pixie.

As we left the room Sally was just shaking her head.

"I simply can't believe it. I've never seen a doctor go for anyone in the way he did with you. I just don't believe it." She went on to explain that there was another option to explore but we would have to "seek leave to appeal." In time they would refuse it but that would not be the end of the story. They gave no reasons for their decision at all and subsequently their decision was overturned at a higher level. That though, was in the future.

The effect on me was devastating. I had been judged, and I had been judged a complete liar. When Sally dropped me back at the house the effects were immediately compounded by my mother. When I told her I'd lost the case she responded with a simple sentence: "I'm not surprised, you made it all up anyway." That was precisely why I hadn't wanted her involved in the first place. Later that evening as I reflected it was clear that it was the most difficult day of my life. Liar, liar. Their judgement. Liar. It disappeared in a haze of smoke. That was the only way to mask the despair, the pain, and the intensity of that voice. But it was back the next day. And the one after that.

The response from the others was very different. The new throngs of people just seemed to accept me and support me even though they were unaware of how grave the situation was. I was just one of them now, living at least partially in reality. That was just as valuable as the hash. Each helped me to get through the day. They didn't judge me although I was always aware that there probably others out there who just dismissed me as a nutter. I was in my language but not in theirs. Throughout that summer I never heard anything derogatory although I found out many years later that some were.

Beyond my immediate problems, there was much going on in the world that summer. The trial of OJ Simpson had been going on for what seemed to be an eternity and was the topic of many a conversation. Most of those joining such conversations felt he was guilty as sin. Western Europe was still trying to figure out and respond to the devastating massacre at a once unknown place called Srebrenica. Yet still we waited for that response. Genocide was reaching what we thought was its full horrors in Europe. We were wrong on that one. There also seemed to be a lot of random murders of young women and girls that summer. Each brought more lurid headlines in the tabloids, but nothing in comparison to the alleged deeds of the now deceased Fred. Another suicide but one that was celebrated rather than mourned by most. His plump wife was still in jail awaiting trial.

As July turned to August I was still reeling form that day at the tribunal. By day I clung desperately to life, by night I got away. But I faced another of my dates that littered my year. The second week in August brought the anniversary of the overdose. Like that day in June, it was another nightmare. With that came greater attempts to run; each worked only until the morning. It had been an enormously difficult couple of months in one respect. In another it had been wonderful. That paradox again. And still they rallied round. August also meant another birthday. Unbeknown to me, life was about to change, and change for the better.

Word filtered out about my birthday but there was another one to get through first. A small gathering took place at the pub at the bottom of the hill exactly one week before I turned twenty six. It was the usual fare, then a retirement to what we anticipated to be an empty house into which one of our company was about to move. We went on late and a handful of us stayed over expecting a late rise followed by a lazy day. I slept soundly in a comfortable bed upstairs. I was rudely awakened alarmingly early by an unknown female voice downstairs. I tried to go back to sleep but failed. The door opened.

"Who the fuck are you and what the fuck are you doing in my bed?" said the unknown voice as I tried to focus from an abrupt awakening. "Where is Pete?"

"I've no idea" I replied, "he was here when we crashed out." Then she disappeared downstairs. It was the ex wife come back to what was supposed to be an empty former residence. When she did catch up with him later I'm told she found it quite funny. Not really what I expected that early in the morning. It was one of the stranger moments of that epic summer. But I was about to have a very strange week.

It was the week that decisive military action was taken by the noble guardians of Western freedom in Bosnia. That combined with the Croatian counter offensive brought all sides to negotiate and effectively ended the terrible genocide that had afflicted so many for so long within a few days. We merely questioned why it had taken so long. Sadly it would not be the end of the catastrophe that had engulfed the Balkans throughout the decade of the 1990s. I'd spent a very pleasant day in Yugoslavia in 1989. Happier days. It was of course impossible to imagine how much things had changed even through the real time of camera.

I was unaware that a plan had been hatched much closer to home some to time earlier that summer. It was revealed to me that week, between the two birthdays. Quietly and unobtrusively my parents had been working behind the scenes again. They had been on holiday some weeks before; as ever I had gone elsewhere for the duration. Ever since we had moved to that small seaside Kent town, my mum had been able to indulge in her passion of swimming. Winter did not keep her out of the sea as long as it was calm. In the early years I used to swim too but my trip to Hong Kong some years before and its warm balmy seas had put paid to my seaside indulgence. After that I'd always thought that she was mad. But she liked it and felt better for it. As a result it was always a stipulation of their rare holidays that she had access to a pool. The last time had been no different.

I took very little notice of what they were saying as they told me this seemingly inane story, but there was a point to it. Whilst there they had become friendly with a fellow bather; and she had a story to tell. She too had a son, a little older than me who had a severe mental illness. He differed from me in a very profound way; he had recovered. He had had the help of a person who described himself simply as a healer. It had taken a long time but it had worked. As they left she had given them a number to call.

My interest was only partially spurred. It sounded like a load of old bollocks but when one is desperate, is there anything to lose? On their return they had called the number.

"We've found the number of a woman in Canterbury and spoken to her. If you want to give it a try, you need to call her." I pondered for a short while. Thoughts kept coming. Bollocks. How can she help me? There is nothing to lose. There were a large number of sceptical thoughts but by that stage I was willing to try anything. I still had my fear of phones so that worried me but I agreed to do it.

I didn't phone straight away as I had to psyche myself up for such action. But I forced myself to do it. She sounded very pleasant on the phone. She suggested we meet for an initial consultation the day after my birthday. Having a vague idea of how I would be feeling I asked to meet a few days after the event. That was my first contact with Caroline. I had no idea just what an impact she would make on my life. All I had was hopelessness, desperation and cynicism.

For most of my life birthdays had been a very lonely experience. I'd boarded since I was nine years old. August was a horrible time to have a birthday if one had no friends at home. I'd had three birthdays on tour and that was the last time that I'd had anything resembling a party. On my fourteenth birthday we were at a post concert reception with the Governor General of Australia. For some reason I'd been conned into speaking, something I apparently pulled off with some aplomb. But that was a long time ago and it hadn't really been personal. This year though things looked different. There were friends and many had said they would come down. We arranged to carry on after the pub at the same house as before, although this time there was no danger of ex wives freaking me out at 9 o' clock in the morning. But I had no knowledge of what other arrangements had been made. As I headed off down the hill early in the evening I was heading into the unknown.

It started off slowly sat at a single table at the back of the garden. Then it snowballed. They came by the dozen. They came from the twilight world of madness and they came from the light filled world of reality. They brought their friends and they brought their families. The young, the old; the unknown and the familiar. As more and more came, so did more tables. And on those tables came more beer. There were presents, both fun and useful. Still they came. There were five tables all connected before we ran out of room. Then it was the ground. Others who were just in the pub came over. Everyone knew someone. Sadly there were a few absentees, the still guarded Jayne and the eccentric artist Beka, but they were few and far between.

As I sat there with this massive throng of happy humanity I had the same thought running through my head. I can't believe they've come for my birthday. They're here for me. It was so new to my life. There were no voices, they had been swiftly neutralised. It didn't even matter that I had to wake up to my mad world the next day. In fact there was no thought of the next day. I was living in the present and not worrying about the future. For one night only I came alive again. But there was more to come.

When the pub shut a number, although not all of us, cabbed it back to the site of the previous week's gathering. I wandered in and turned to the right into the small living room just inside the door. I was confronted by a small yet excitable dog that ran and leapt about to greet the visitors. I went to sit down but Laura stopped me.

"What are you doing?"
"I'm sitting down."
"We're not here, we're upstairs." I was mystified. It would have been hard enough to fit us all in downstairs but I couldn't envisage gathering upstairs. "Come up" she said. I followed her and Pete up the stairs. As we got to the top I saw a lowered ladder leading to a hatch to the loft. It was narrow, steep and moderately alarming considering our communal state of drunkenness. I climbed carefully and slowly. There in front was a loft space covering the entire size of the admittedly small house. All around the edges were cushions

and mattresses. A stereo had been set up as had a TV. I was stunned. It turned out that they had spent all afternoon preparing for the evening. I had been both struck and moved by everyone's generosity and care in my honour for turning up. They were there for me, a feeling I'd rarely had in my life. And now this.

The loft was soon full of about fifteen people, all comfortably sat in the eaves of the house. There were bottles and cans. The air was quickly awash with smoke. Some I knew, some I didn't. But it didn't matter. An absent friend who lived over the road came to investigate the noise and quickly joined us. The mad, the sane, the old, the young. There were no barriers that night. We were united in a desire to celebrate. Celebrate my birthday. Then my disbelief was stretched even further. Laura produced a decorated chocolate birthday cake. This led to the slightly alarming sight of James wandering around the small loft wielding a carving knife. Sadly, most of us were too stoned to manage the dryness of cake but I was overwhelmed by everyone's effort.

As night moved towards day, some drifted off home. Others fell where they sat. One was so sound asleep we wondered whether he was still alive. Many years later, on a very difficult Christmas day, he came up to me in the pub and reminded me of that day. I was amazed that he remembered who I was.

Around dawn I finally relented to the need for sleep. I overcame my night long fear of someone falling through the hatch and gingerly moved down to a sofa in the front room. I slept the sleep of the contented that night, with not a thought of the pain of the morning. I knew it would be there but it didn't matter. The pain had gone for now.

I can never remember when summer finishes and autumn starts. I don't suppose it matters really, but in my eyes autumn starts with the arrival of September. With that comes the NFL season and a few other hours of respite each week. That party marked the end of an extraordinary summer. I'd met so many people and they were real, not in the shadows like my other people. The little pub at the bottom of the hill that I had feared so much had become almost my second home. It was in fact the zenith for the place, it was great the next summer but it never was the same. Within three years it had almost died. For many months after people I'd never met talked about wishing they had been at the party. Most of us had fond memories.

I had gained a toehold in reality that summer. But by day it was different. The night was a distraction but I would always wake up in the morning. I was still ill. Life was both desperate and hopeless. I could still travel, and there were now new places to go. The itinerancy of my madness went on.

A couple of days into September not much had really changed. Maybe there was hope in this healer. Scepticism still reigned in my world though.

Chapter 21

The Leaping Dog

I've never liked dogs. Dirty, noisy, smelly, slobbery things. The misfortune of treading in their remnants walking along the pavements. The way they jump up at people and lick them. The drool they seem to produce. I've never found any feature of canine behaviour remotely attractive. Not only do I dislike them, I distrust them too. The common call of "it won't bite" never held any water in my eyes. Unpredictable. What I do understand though is people's need and desire to have pets, be they canine or feline. There's something unconditional about them. They depend on and use their owners but they are on the whole deeply affectionate. Companions for the lonely and the loved at the same time. I grew up around cats. At the time of my descent into madness we had two cats. Within days of the start that number had been reduced to one. It was the third of the traumas of that week; maybe bad news does come in threes. The survivor though was one of the most affectionate creatures one could ever come across. He was ginger, had giant feet, and was very stupid. His feet, with an extra toe on each paw gave away his presence as he got hitched in the carpet when he approached. Through much of my illness, especially when I was at my worst, he seemed to be my only link to reality, a little anchor point on the edge of the swamp into which I was drowning.

Over the years I'd had many friends with dogs, and, although I still disliked and distrusted them, I had learned to tolerate them. That was the price I paid for all my travelling. They were an irritant to me but I had had to put up with them. Most people blamed the owners for the misfortune heaped at the door of dogs, but dog shit is still dog shit when one steps in it. They also talked about training frequently but even with those that were well trained, my tolerance was tempered by that distrust. Most of the time though, I didn't really think about dogs if I could possibly help it.

Dogs were the last thing on my mind as I drove once again into the unknown on the road to Canterbury. I was much more concerned about finding the house of this mysterious woman who described herself merely as a "healer". One rather peculiar, and unexplained, feature of my illness was a complete loss of any sense of direction. Driving or walking to new places always raised my anxiety levels. I would also get very anxious about being on time. I had directions but I didn't trust my senses at all. Canterbury is not a particularly good place to get around by car. Looking at the map, the route took me in a completely different direction to my previously known experience. Then there were the one way roads and the cul de sacs. That's where I ran into difficulties. Amid much panic I did get there eventually, not so fashionably late.

I knocked tentatively on a brightly coloured door. As it swung open I was confronted by a beaming woman in her thirties who invited me in. The interior was also strikingly bright with a radiance to it. That radiance reflected in her too. She just seemed to have an aura of good surrounding her, an aura extending from that broad smile. Here was a professional, a very different professional. I could not tell what it was about her but she exuded positivity from almost every pore. She invited me into the front room. It was light and warm with a massage table to one side. The walls were adorned with a variety of Buddhist imagery but it didn't give off a sense of being a religious place; iconography I could deal with, religion I could not. We sat opposite one another in wicker chairs and just began to talk. She took some brief details, pondered for a while and told me it would take more than a few sessions. That though, was nothing new to me. The talking was easy just like two old friends meeting up for the first time in a while. There were no boundaries or the usual stand off of those I'd met before. There was connection there, and that was new. Within minutes she had taught me to breathe properly. That may not seem very important but in all the years of singing no one had managed to teach me that. She talked about the ability of animals to sense us and our vibes. That didn't really seem to be very important at the time either and actually fed my scepticism a little. But the scepticism was slipping away.

She taught me to visualise in but a few minutes. I felt a modicum of calm come over me with that. Time shifted in that room. Shifting time had been a very uncomfortable experience of my illness but there was a great stillness here. It was just comfortable in that light and airy room. After a time that seemed immeasurable she asked me to lie face down on the massage table. Things got very strange then. I could feel her move around me and sense the nearness of her hands yet there was no contact. As I lay there, a calm descended in a way I'd never known before. There was no physical sensation at all just a sensory change. Not only was it calming it was relaxing. Peace was descending on my troubled mind. I was sleepy but not sleepy. Calm.

I've no idea how long it went on for but when she'd finished I felt like a different person. Not as I'd been before the madness but different. I paid my money and arranged to come back the next week. As I drove home I tried to reflect on the experience but could make nothing of it. All I knew was that I felt better and realised I'd stumbled across something very significant. I just couldn't place exactly what it was. But this was relief without the use of foreign substances. That relief lasted about half an hour.

Within days of this first meeting I was back on my travels again. Ros had been there for me since the early days and I still had an invitation to visit when I wanted. It was a different world in Wimbledon, but still my world followed. Ros was one of my friends with a dog. When I arrived, the elderly Ryan had seen better days and spent most of his time curled up on the sofa. He rarely moved unless he had to; when he did, he more or less crawled everywhere. His youthful exuberance, similar to that of most canine creatures had gone. I'd been there for a couple of days when I decided to try the visualisation that Caroline had taught me. Taking my leave and explaining that I would be about twenty minutes, I headed upstairs to lie down. With my concentration still very weak it took some time to focus. It was much harder on my own but I did manage to get through it. There was the merest hint of a brief spark in my mind but the effects were very short.

When I'd finished, I went back down the stairs. As I walked through the kitchen to the conservatory where they were all sitting, Ryan leapt up off the sofa. He ran towards me. The others looked on stunned. When he got to me he started to circle me and leap up as young dogs are wont to do. None of us knew what was going on, what to do, or indeed to say. With Ryan still leaping Ros broke the collective silence.

"What the fuck have you done to the dog?"

"I've no idea." As I spoke, Caroline's words about animals came back into my mind. Something had happened. I didn't know what it was but I did know that it very real and palpable. It was then that I realised the power she possessed. To this day neither she nor I know how it works but it does. Ryan did eventually exhaust himself and retire again to the sofa. And I started to believe. The rest of my stay was uneventful.

My parents paid for the first few sessions with her and I went weekly or fortnightly through September. But cost would be an issue in the future. I'd found a treatment that worked for me, albeit for only a short period of time, but that was better than anything else I had tried or experienced. When I told my GP of its effectiveness he looked into getting it funded by his practice. She had two feeder surgeries in Canterbury but sadly the partners where I went refused to do so. Although I needed it more frequently I had to settle on going once a month. Heather helped once again when she was able to secure six months funding from the National Schizophrenia Fellowship. I had supporters but sadly those with the real power and influence weren't very interested. The bottom line though was that once a month there was a tiny glimmer of hope and relief; and that was priceless.

In the real world significant legal cases were about to follow one another on both sides of the Atlantic. The lengthy proceedings against OJ Simpson for double murder reached their zenith that autumn. Much to the shock of many throughout the world he was acquitted. Expensive lawyers seemed to have won the day in the face of overwhelming odds. Who knows the truth, but most were left in a state of disbelief. Within days though he had been all but forgotten in this country as the plump wife of the man called Fred went on trial for multiple murders.

In the days that followed the public and perhaps more significantly the tabloids were transfixed by events at Winchester Crown Court. Day after day more and more gory details filled our papers. Horror and fascination became unusual bed fellows as events unfurled. Perhaps most shocking was the death mask of a fifteen year old girl who's young, smiling, and slightly shy face appeared most days along with those of the other victims. It was almost unspeakable;

and that was only what was reported. Much was left in the court room.

Rose denied any knowledge of what went on in that small, scruffy house in Gloucester's bed-sit land. In her defence she simply blamed Fred. He had admitted his guilt before his death but he wasn't there to face the charges. The jury refused to believe her and found her guilty of murder ten times over. She was sentenced to a corresponding number of life sentences. Later she would be told that she would never be released. The last great, sensational "trial of the century" as the tabloids dubbed it in the United Kingdom of the twentieth century was over. The fall out and the subsequent books would last for some to come. I was still an avid reader of the genre. Some were truly horrifying but yet again who knew the real truth of what had happened? Only Rose now held those secrets.

Whilst my visits to leafy Wimbledon were comparatively rare, journeys to more salubrious parts of south London were much more commonplace. Throughout that autumn and early winter I regularly travelled to Bermondsey, and to Borough, and to Elephant and Castle. It was a world far removed from the now no longer quiet seaside town in Kent that was the place of my residence. The streets felt much less safe, with the night time drinking trips on the Old Kent Road verging on the scary. All around was deprivation, poverty, drugs, violence, racism, alcoholism, and for many fear of the National Front. Yet there were wonderful people there who each and every day struggled for survival. All my friends from the Hotel were always welcoming and pleased to see me. We'd gather in one flat or another, reminisce and try to forget our similar problems. We made a strange group, so different in our backgrounds yet drawn so closely together by ill health. They like all those I'd met on journey, were what kept me going. We partied hard but we had much to forget. I met others through them, the neighbours with different but equally devastating problems. Seeing some of them gave me a flicker of hope as they gave up the fight and retreated into a bottle far larger than I could even pick up. Sadly, I'm sure some of them are no longer with us. They, like all the others, accepted me into that world. I'd been thrown in there almost by mistake, but so many riches were to be found in such desolation.

A Pillar of Impotence

As a result of my many forays to London, in December I received a second invite to the Hotel Christmas party. Normally former patients were invited back the year they had left, but the regularity of my visits to old friends elicited an unusual further invite. It was always good to see my people but on this occasion there was the disadvantage of meeting god again. Whilst I knew he would be both polite and pleased to see me, he would inevitably judge me. That was a great fear. As I'd always said none of us could ever leave the Hotel, and his judgement followed us all. It was a fear that I talked to Caroline about and she suggested another form of visualisation specifically for him. I was unconvinced though.

Following the form of the previous year, the first part in the ward would be low key. Then, those of us who could, would head across the small courtyard to the pub that fronted onto the main road. I was extremely nervous when I arrived, even though I was fortified by a quick visit to the pub first. There he was with his smiling, friendly face on, oozing that charm that I'd seen the first time I had met him, and smoking his ultra light cigarettes. Much as I wanted to avoid him he did seek me out. No obvious judgement but I could feel him inside. We talked as he enquired how I was. Then it happened.

"Have you got a plan?" The memory of our last conversation before my departure kept coming into my thoughts. Whatever you do, there must be a purpose to it. Whatever you do, there must be a purpose to it. Over it came as I stumbled to think of an answer.
"I was thinking of looking into going back to Cambridge to do a PGCE." It just slipped off my tongue without even thinking what I had said.
"I'm sure they'd let you do that. I think it's a good idea." What have I let myself in for? I have to justify myself. He's judging me again. Then I tried to kick in with the visualisation. Much to my surprise, it seemed to work. For a brief while I lost his conversation. It didn't matter. As he moved away to talk to others, he just drifted off out of my life; at least for the time being.

The rest of the night was the usual fair of most of my trips to the capital. Pub; flat; smoke; and drink. On we went into the oblivion of another night. We all expected the pain to return in the morning.

I never saw god again after that night. But the memory of our brief conversation stuck with me. What had come from me had surprised me and had been merely an effort to stop him judging me; I had also unwittingly laid down a challenge to myself. I had often in my lonely musings thought about that final lost year in Cambridge. Sometimes it felt as if Cambridge somehow owed me a year. The place had always been what I considered to be my real home and I had an overwhelming desire to go home one day. But how? A PGCE had been muted by those in the know many times before but it seemed an impossibility, the pipedream of a madman that would always remain just that. I simply wasn't well enough. Neither did I have the means, method or support to even think about trying. Yet I had still challenged myself.

The Christmas holidays brought everyone back to the seaside and the parties started again. As usual at that time of year though, I became much more unstable. Christmas always brought extra pain.

They celebrated New Year too; I just drank to forget. Yet each morning it all came back. In January my future was still very uncertain. I had Caroline and the brief relief after her sessions but I couldn't see beyond that half hour, one hour, or, if lucky, two hours that was my calm. Real long term hope still eluded me as my head pounded and the voices and music interrupted so many of my waking moments.

Chapter 22

Not at Work Today Then?

Education held onto me for much of my early life. It had been a privileged background in many respects, but it was privilege secured mainly by my ability to sing not by my family's ability to pay for it. I'd travelled the world at an early age, met many distinguished people, and sat through more recording sessions than I care to remember. On the whole, recording is a tedious and painstaking process; the buzz often only comes at the end. Music had been my means into Cambridge and all the decadence, pomp, and often arrogance that the institution affords. Cambridge also offered rich rewards, both financial and cultural. I had foolishly spurned most of the latter. As for work and remuneration, that had been swept away by circumstance.

In the late winter of 1996 I was almost five years removed from the education that was supposed to have set me up for life. Those so terribly affected by the recession were mainly over it. All my friends had jobs and were leading successful lives; I was drifting and still in pain. Nothing had changed much and little was forthcoming from those trained to deal with the likes of me. I still took my pills, but, sleep apart, they did nothing for me. There was nothing new on offer. My symptoms were the same and no one seemed to have any solution. Not only that, those who knew didn't seem to believe a word I said. The Evil Pixie had left to great rejoicing among the brethren. Her replacement was a quiet, slight, and kindly man. He was very different to the others I'd met over the years; he seemed to actually care. That said though, he appeared to have no more of idea where to go next than anyone else. Caroline did help but the effects of her amazing and strange treatment were, like the effects of the weed of the evening, limited; they wore off quickly. In the world of confidentiality I was going nowhere. In the real world it was getting harder.

People have told me that I have always looked younger than I actually am. In my teens I'd hated that. From about eighteen onwards it hadn't really mattered, I could legally drink. Through my early to mid twenties everyone always assumed that I was a student.

No real need to justify my existence. Justification and judgement seemed a universal fear amongst my people. Prove one's ill health to the DSS. Hide one's ill health from those who enquired how one managed to get such a nice flat. That one didn't worry me but it did others. Where do you get your money from? Another question for those who were lucky enough not to have been screwed as badly by the DSS as I had been. What do you do for a living? It was a question I faced on occasions and usually squirmed before being brutally honest; many assumed I was bullshitting with my answer. We all feared those questions.

As the winter of my twenty seventh year passed the pretence or assumption of studentship had more or less gone. The disadvantage of now knowing so many more people, not only people in my world but those in the world of reality, was that the questions became more and more frequent. Justify. Justify. Prove your worth in society. And that added to the anxiety and pain.

Being something of a creature of habit I've been going to the same place to get my hair cut since moving to Kent. I must have been about ten when I first walked into the little shop in the middle of the high street of the small and insignificant town that was my part time residence, if not in my eyes my home. They were very friendly in there and seemed to deal with my wild and notoriously curly hair okay. As I entered the second half of my twenties it had become a much more frightening place. Every time I entered and sat in the chair I was greeted in the same way.

"Not at work today then?" It was of course a very simple comment that was just intended to start the sort of small talk the English are renowned for. But for me it was a very direct assault. What do I say? Why have I come? Why do they want to know? They're not really interested. Justify yourself. However prepared I was my mind always exploded in a plethora of thoughts. I'd shake just a little more. I'd tense up and start to sweat. The physical pain would increase. Run! Get out! But I couldn't. I'd just mumble whatever came into my head then sit in silence as they cut and moved. I often wondered what they must make of me but never came up with an answer.

A Pillar of Impotence

It would have been easier if the conversation stayed there though. Often it didn't. Many are condemnatory of those who don't work and claim from the state. That wonderfully strange concept, the Australian soap opera that had been introduced to us in the eighties had even brought a title for us; dole bludger. They'd brought the word Uni. too, an immensely cultural enrichment of our world. Such people seemed to be a favourite topic of conversation for those who worked in the barbers when they unable to engage the customer in any meaningful type of conversation. Often they talked of this person or that and accused them of laziness, or fraud, or commented that there was nothing wrong with them. Each word added to my discomfort. It was usually a relief to get out. I did think about going elsewhere but always imagined that it would be the same anywhere. These were the barbs that the mad had to endure in so many areas of their lives. So many feared the mentally ill because they knew nothing about them. And so often we can't see madness, we merely suffer it.

Not much changed that spring. Once a month I visited Caroline. I went to the pub at the bottom of the hill. I drank and I smoked to dull the pain. I struggled for sleep aided only by the chemicals I swallowed at night. I fought on every day without purpose. My mood moved up and down in its subterranean lift for no apparent reason. I waited for news on my DLA. Every now and then a great missive would arrive through the post; for some obscure reason copies of everything were sent each time. I now had a mountain of paper stashed away. And I travelled.

It was also in the spring that I travelled on one of my regular trips to London. Although I disliked the place it was the people who made the visits worthwhile. On this occasion I stayed with an old friend from the Hotel in a small tower block close to Elephant and Castle. Although it was relatively friendly in that block, the area was often dangerous and hostile with elements of a ghetto mentality all around. Like so many such places it was, to an extent, a dumping ground for the poor, the oppressed, and the vulnerable. The failure of Care in the Community had been wreaked there. I was a regular visitor there but this occasion would be different. This time I was meeting up with Rachel. Although we were in regular touch, I had not seen her for some time. She had been in London since the previous autumn, but, despite my frequent visits to the city, we had not, as yet, met up there.

It was warm and sunny the day that we met. We returned to one of our old haunts from my days in the Hotel. As ever it was an amiable meeting as we sipped cold drinks on the banks of the Thames. There was no hint of change, no rejection, the one thing I feared most from our meetings. As ever the mask that had descended across her mind so long ago was up. The usual religious undertones still existed which served only as a mild irritant to an otherwise pleasant day. Much as I loved to see Rachel there was always an element of anxiety on my part. That had been there since the madness descended on me. Under that lay fear but our conversations never went that deep; they were always guarded on both of our parts. To those around us we were just a pair of people meeting for a drink. Nothing gave away the enormity of the past as we both skirted around things, the depth of that past had long since gone.

When we parted and headed to our respective transportation my thoughts were tinged with a mix of sadness and exhaustion. It had been a meeting like so many we had had before. We would continue to stay in touch and meet again soon. As I walked back to the Elephant nothing seemed to have changed, I just needed to de-stress for a while and I had some excellent wares back at the flat for just such an eventuality. I was blissfully unaware that that would prove to be our final meeting. It was the last time I would see that haunting face. The finality would only hit much later.

Back at the flat I rolled a large spliff. There was both relief and sadness going through my mind as I sat on the sofa and lit it. My host pottered around doing various household things, pausing briefly and occasionally to take a few hits. I mused on the religious elements of my meeting very relieved that they were over. As I sat in a haze of smoke there was a knock at the door.

"Can you get that?" said a disembodied voice delivered form the vicinity of the kitchen.
"No problem." I crossed the short distance, spliff in hand, cutting my way through the dense smoke to the door. Turning the Yale lock I pulled the door open expecting to see familiar faces come to join us. There before me stood two middle aged men, smartly dressed

and holding a sheaf of magazines and a couple of small books. What the fuck are they doing here? For a split second I was stumped as I marvelled at the beautiful but bright red tie around the neck of the closest man to me. He had a large moustache. As soon as he opened his mouth I knew who they were. Brave men come to do the Lord's work. The smoke blew out of the door towards them, driven on by the breeze from an open window behind me, a legacy of a fine, warm spring day. The spliff hung unsmoked between the fingers of my left hand; I didn't notice when it went out naturally. More religion. Thoughts.

Unlike many others I'm never rude to the messengers of Jehovah. I listened politely as they ran off their routine. I had no interest in it, but neither had I any interest in stopping them from doing what they felt they had to do; we are all entitled to our beliefs. What I had a problem with was their belief that they were right and everyone else was wrong. I'd had that that afternoon already. I don't know how long it was before they left but I suspect it was longer than they would spend with most of their hosts for the rest of the afternoon. I accepted a copy of their magazine and they headed off up the stairs. I admired their bravery if not their beliefs. They were brave men indeed to try to spread their message in that place.

It had been a strangely if not entirely unexpected religious day. As I relit the remnants of the dwindling spliff, those thoughts remained for some time, even in oblivion.

The lighter days of spring and early summer always caused me problems. I was still afflicted by intense head and eye pain. The longer hours of light and sun served to exacerbate that condition. Still I wore shades for most of my waking outdoor hours. It also heralded that anniversary in the middle of June, the death of my old life and the start of my living death. I'd long since stopped going to the hidden place by the water's edge. I'd also stopped listening to much of my music. It just caused too much pain. But the music went on when I was at my worst. In fact the psychotic mental jukebox was the normal precursor to coming pain. It always started the same. The notes and songs were initially quiet, distant, and detached. Yet as I descended the volume increased. Then it became random. My subconscious brought back complete and long forgotten melodies and lines at deafening levels. I never really escaped the music in my head, the songs that had been woven into the fabric of my madness. It terrified me. Yet I started to make it deliberately more painful. I'd met many people on my journey who cut themselves. Initially most were victims of voices telling them to do it. At the Hotel there were others, those who sought relief from their mental pain or merely to punish themselves further. Cutting to kill was rare in my experience. I never cut myself physically I just did it mentally. I would deliberately go to the most painful places and listen to the most painful music when I was at my worst. Anything to increase the pain and punish. I was piece of shit and I deserved to suffer further. Mental cutting, another of the paradoxes of madness. I did it in the middle of June when I expected to be bad. For all the good that had happened in the last year, I still suffered, and I still did it. Summer was here, as were the students. Three months of parties beckoned but still I wrestled my demons. And no one could do anything about it. That was my life. In mid June I knew it was coming, at other times I didn't; the madness remained random.

Whilst the pain and instability of mid June was the norm, much of the rest of that summer was shaping up to be decidedly abnormal. I hadn't been on a summer choir trip since I was fourteen. My most recent trips had always been at Easter, and I'd not been on one of those for three years. One was in the planning stages when I was in the Hotel but it failed to materialise. I was relieved in a slightly selfish way. Memories of the trip to Prague had also influenced thinking and made everyone a little wary of touring again. This year it was different. An invitation had been secured to spend a week as a visiting choir at Chartres. This was a departure from our usual format which was rather more relaxed and took in a number of different venues. I had my usual reservations and fears. I was very concerned about the schedule and questioned whether I had the stamina to manage that amount of singing any more. But on the whole I was looking forward to it, and that was very much a departure from my usual state of mind. It was little target for me, the future and not the past.

There was also the prospect of the country hosting the *Euro 96* tournament. No one could have possibly predicted the phenomenon that it would create. Over a period of a couple of weeks the whole country seemed to be galvanised and uplifted in their support of England. A tremendous feel good factor gripped us all in a way I'd not seen since the euphoria of the Gulf War all those years before. People seemed to be genuinely united in their support and in their Englishness. First the old Scots enemy was slain. Then the shock of hammering the Dutch. We were buzzing. The Spanish too were deposed in a rather closer run battle. Then of course it all went wrong. Germany. The bubble burst. Violence. I was glad I wasn't in London that day. I watched the final with Trapper but we weren't really very interested at that stage. For a couple of weeks our world changed. It was indeed a strange summer.

It's not often that events beyond our control have a real impact on our lives. *Euro 96* had had an impact but it wasn't really anything more than an impact of perception. It was an event much closer to home, a much darker one, that really impacted on my life although the significance would not become clear until two years later.

It was on a July afternoon not too far up the road from the little seaside town that a mother, her two young daughters and their dog set off across the fields for home after a swimming gala. By all accounts it was not a long walk for them. On their journey they encountered another person, probably a man. After an unknown amount of time the mother, the youngest daughter, and the dog lay dead, bludgeoned with a blunt instrument, probably a hammer. Josie, the elder of the two was left for dead. In fact when the family was found it was thought that she too was dead. Somehow she survived. It was indeed a black July day.

There was a great deal of unease in the local community. It was too close to home and there was an unknown killer loose in that community. In the underworld in which I lived part of my life, the world of the mentally ill, there was even more consternation. We all knew or suspected that whoever had done such a shocking deed would be, or would claim to be one of us. More headlines, more stigma. When a man was put on trial two years later he would change the world of the mad. More legislation would be promised.

There was another tragedy that July. An airliner exploded over the Atlantic, not far from the coast of the United States. Terrorism was immediately suspected. As I waited for the days to pass away before my trip, we all still lived in very uncertain times.

Chapter 23

Psychotic Zadok

Few people around the local area wanted it but they built it anyway. The great project to connect us to continental Europe had been met with widespread scepticism in the towns on the Kent coast. Traders feared that the Channel Tunnel would move visitors out and on before they could spend any of their hard earned cash in the coastal town. Ashford would get the grand title of Ashford International at its station and a potential boom; the coast faced decay and deprivation. Travellers would be whisked there and to London without delay. There was a great deal of political will behind the idea but no government finance. For years we faced the eye sore of construction, of fields gauged out and turned into a sea of mud. Houses had to be compulsorily purchased, the rugby club was moved, and there were lurid stories of people being forced to sell their land for a pittance. It was not popular. It was very much a paradox economically in the area. In the short and medium term there were employment opportunities in its construction, but in the longer term the downturn of being sidelined. It brought many new people to the area for a while, then, when it was complete, they moved on. It did create jobs in the Duty Free areas but that too would be swept away in time as we came closer to Europe. We didn't want it but it had been a reality for two years by the summer of 1996. And that would be my means to my next musical end.

Although I had been looking forward to the trip for some time, I was much more nervous than on previous such events. Whilst the Tunnel itself held no fears for me the crowds that would inevitably await me in the Paris Metro were another story. The panic I felt in crowds had long afflicted me to such an extent that I hadn't set foot in a supermarket in about five years. Although I regularly used the London Underground, I had the luxury of at least knowing where I was going there. The faster I got out of a crowd the better and that seemed less likely to happen with a large group of people on unfamiliar territory. The travel time to Paris would be relatively quick but getting across the city and then catching another train to the south would make the journey uncomfortably long. Then there was the schedule itself. On paper it looked like the most intense period of sustained singing I had had to endure since childhood. For someone in the permanent state of exhaustion that my illness had bequeathed me it was daunting prospect.

But there was a darker fear within me. I'd always been linguistically challenged. Unlike Miriam who seemed to have a flare for languages I had neither a flare for nor an interest in the words of others. Throughout school I had singularly failed in the field although I did somehow scrape a C in O level French. But that was years before and my linguistic arsenal extended little beyond being able to order a beer abroad and be polite. It had never really been much of an issue on many of my travels but in the weeks leading up to our departure I had a series of disturbing thoughts. For some reason I became convinced that I would get ill in France and be carted off to some French nuthouse where no one would speak English. However much I tried to dismiss them, the thoughts kept coming. They were never strong enough to outweigh the desire to go but they did cast an ominous shadow over the lead up to my first, and so far only trip on the *Eurostar*. Fortunately as I set off for Ashford International on a sunny July day, such thoughts were not overwhelming.

It was always a complex and tedious process transporting forty odd people from one country to another, allocating rooms and getting settled in; it was one I avoided having much to do with if I could. Having arrived at the station, said my hellos to old friends, and passed through the various formalities, I adjourned to the bar to wait. I was pleasantly surprised to see the excellent *Hurlimanns* on offer in cans and enthusiastically introduced the others to a local tradition. The wait was not long and soon we were aboard and headed underground. Being in the tunnel itself was a curious non event; there was no real sense of motion, it merely felt as if someone had turned the light off. It was like the darkness of night for about twenty minutes then the sun came out again. Unlike some of the others in our party the tunnel held no fears for me. The only disturbing aspect of that part of the journey was discovering that *Eurostar* held no licence to sell Duty Free. Whilst the journey was okay I had mounting nerves about the prospect of the Metro.

When we got there after a very pleasant and relaxing ride the Metro proved to be just as bad as I feared. Panic, sweat, fear, confusion. All of these feelings hit me as we tried to work out where we were going. Even aboard the train the crowds and lack of space did nothing to avert my fear and underground there is nowhere to run to. It eased somewhat as we reached our destination and waited for our next train. But by that stage I was getting very weary and with that my mind raced off in a different direction. There was relief when we arrived at Chartres station but it was only a temporary respite as we had a considerable journey on foot, laden with bags to get to our final destination. Shattered, I arrived and then had to wait to get organised. The view of this vast cathedral was a breathtaking backdrop to my wait though. We were quartered in a school right next to the monument to the power and wealth of the mediaeval Catholic Church. Eventually I made it inside and just collapsed on the bed. But that was just part of an already exhausting day. There were rehearsals to conduct after dinner.

Some hours later I was able to finally retire to a bar for some well earned beers. We sat outside the nearest one we could find just across the square from the cathedral. Others fanned out across the city in the traditional search for the best and cheapest bars. It always seems odd to me that our continental brethren allow one to pay at the end, but then I suppose they consider us equally odd for us requiring payment on request. Of course the difficulty of the continental system is that it is harder to know how much things will cost at the end. But we thought little of that as the waiter took our order. Most of us elected for a medium beer, a half litre. One of our company decided to push the boat out and go for the grande option, the full litre. We sat on a warm evening, tired but doing at last what we did best. After one drink we decided to move on and asked for the bill. When it came it was a devastating shock. The half litre was £5, the litre £10. The exchange rate had shafted us. We had walked into a place of exorbitant prices and not many of us had planned for that. We were however all cheered by the comment of the litre man, "I can afford about another nine of those." Fortunately we quickly found a cheaper alternative but not much. It had indeed been a long day.

The first day of trips was always hectic but things usually settled down very quickly. I would just try to switch into choir trip mode and hope that my stamina held out for a week or so. This time though the schedule was relentless. On the Sunday we sang twice in the morning, no time even for a cigarette break. Then again in the afternoon. That was something I'd never done even as a child. When not singing services there were rehearsals. Respite was rare and I'd had almost no time to recover from the travelling. My fears for my mental state grew rapidly, and the prospect of a French nuthouse loomed larger. And being abroad I had no way of keeping the really bad stuff under wraps; the relief of smoking was not an option. Each day we sang and each night we drank and ate. With the passing days the weariness grew both in my mind and my voice. There was one day off and there was a plan to go to *Euro Disney* then. It was not a place I would have chosen to go to but at least it would be a day away from the rigours of the schedule.

But it was not only the itinerary that played on my mind. As ever there were new faces and with them came the potential questions, the eternal need to justify my existence. For the first few days there was nothing, I merely kept up the pretence of being "normal." I regaled people with my many stories and they accepted me. That all changed the night before our free day. It was early in the evening, in one of our regular bars. She sat there drinking cocktails, the daughter of a psychiatrist but I didn't feel threatened. All around us the others were unwinding after another long day. We were just talking when it came out.

"So, what do you do then?" A simple question but not for me. It just came out, the truth.
"I'm a psychiatric patient." She didn't flinch, and just carried on fascinated. We talked with others oblivious. It was easy to get lost in the crowd, just two people having a conversation amidst a large throng. On and on we talked, quietly and unobtrusively. When we moved to the next bar we carried on. Still no one took any notice. Memories of Prague came back, the same connection just different circumstances. She had no need, just a thirst for knowledge from a personification of her father's work. In return I found a rare peace.

As the last bar shut a few of us sat in the square outside the monolith. Spirits were high. The local beggar approached from time to time, requesting money or cigarettes; the last of my *Gauloises* went that way. As the hours moved on towards dawn, the others drifted off. We were alone now and still we talked. Close to dawn we finally gave up the ghost and bowed to the inevitable exhaustion. Tired though I was, the peace had lasted.

It was another early rise the next day. We passed each other over breakfast and she asked if I had any regrets. This rather surprised me but I had none. The theme park was rather better than I had expected although we were completely unable to find a beer. As the day went on though, my stamina was again sapped. It was a day of rest but it still added to my weariness. Towards the end of the afternoon all I could manage was to sit down and rest. My exhaustion was beginning to accumulate alarmingly, and with that my fears grew; choir trip mode was wearing dangerously thin. The following day it was back to the punishing schedule.

We always ended our trips with the Last Supper. There was a particular poignancy to the last night for me; it had after all been on the last night that Rachel had entered my life. It had been just over six years since that had happened; six years and so much pain. In the final run up to that last night we took in Paris by night, an exhilarating yet extraordinarily expensive evening. I'd been there before but my mind was on others things then and I'd completely failed to appreciate it. And then there was the last service which would finish with the great blast that is *Zadok the Priest*. *Zadok*, however, required a fresh and powerful voice. Unfortunately at the end of the most intense period of singing since I was a child, my voice was shot.

Having precariously negotiated most of the service I waited for the organ to herald the finale. For the first couple of bars things seemed very normal, they were bars I'd heard countless times before. Then things went horribly wrong. I heard a voice, a tangible voice. It was high above, echoing around the vast vault of the cathedral. My first thought was that someone had come in the wrong place. But they hadn't. It carried on. Within a few seconds I recognised the voice. It was hers, it was real, and it was outside of my head. Terror gripped me as I shut down from all that was around me. It can't be. She's outside my head. It makes no sense. Stop, please stop! But on it went. There had only been a couple of occasions on which I had heard Rachel's voice outside my head and they had been only single sentences. But it wasn't just the fact that I was hearing it that was odd and alarming, it was the structure of the music itself. The opening choral lines were in perfect harmony with the organ introduction. That can't happen. It's wrong. Thoughts came very fast but the voice didn't stop. Run. You can't run. You've never run. You're in a cathedral. I'd run once before in Prague but that had been easier, there was no congregation to pass through there. No one must know. No one must know. Hide. But there was nowhere to hide. "Zadok the priest and Nathan the prophet anointed Solomon king" screamed the voice. Then it went on. "And all the people rejoiced." It shouldn't fit cried my thought. But it does come to the mental riposte.

As the organ got louder as it headed for the real choral entrance, her voice crescendoed with it. Still the impossible was happening, the harmony was perfect. I could sense my eyes narrowing as they were wont to do when I had my attacks. All around the others waited in anticipation unaware of the battle going on within and without my head. I was no longer in touch with anything around me, I was just getting by on auto pilot. The terror increased as the organ thundered towards the dramatic entry of the choir. Then the cathedral exploded with sound and her voice was gone. Gone from the atmosphere but not from my head. Internally a torrent of sound engulfed me. She was having her vengeance.

I made it through without running. As we processed out her voice, the man's voice yelling "time to die", and my thoughts fought a constant battle. With the thoughts of others turning to the forthcoming party I stepped outside, still robed, and lit a cigarette. Almost motionless I stared into space, moving only to draw on the cigarette. I was trying to work out what to do to stop it. Visions of the French nuthouse crowded in, jostling for position with the other thoughts and the voices. What I needed was a spliff but that was not going to happen.

Out of the corner of my eye I became aware of one of the girls standing a few feet away from me.

"Are you alright?" I think that's what she said but I could not respond. Get the fuck out of my space. You're intruding. But I could not respond either verbally or by looking at her. It was my private hell and no one was allowed in such moments of despair. Then she moved away and let me be.

When I eventually left the cathedral for the last time I resolved to return to the school to take a shower and get away from everyone else. It was deserted when I got there. Voices still raging, I stepped into the shower, shut the door, and turned the water on. That's when it got even worse. The walls and door started to cave in on me in a crushing movement. I'd never hallucinated visually, and, fortunately, never have since. At the same time the voices were screaming. I tried to scream but nothing came out. No one would have heard even if I had made a noise. I was alone and in sheer terror. Still the walls kept coming in but never touching me. What little was left of my conscious mind fought but it didn't stop. I got out as fast as I could.

As I dressed I feared the rest of the night. I was in my paradox, I craved to be alone but had a desperate need to be with others. Being with others was inevitable though, there was a party to attend. There seemed only one way to try to alleviate the pain: to get as pissed as I could possibly get and hope that the voices would stop.

Through most of the early evening I was quiet and sullen. Dinner passed with no alleviation of symptoms. All around the others celebrated the end of another successful trip; I stared into space speaking only when it was necessary. In the bar I quietly drank hoping that it would get easier. We followed our habit of starting in one particular bar, a habit honed over the week by the lack of resources of most of us. And then the change came. As my alcohol levels increased I woke from my mental slumber and began to live again. The more I drank the more the voices diminished. I started to talk and the psychiatrist's daughter was there for me. We moved on to next bar that would be our final stop off point. The hours drifted on. My exhaustion disappeared along with the voices and I was back to life, the man they all expected.

When the bar closed we carried on in the square. As it got colder we moved indoors. Dawn was coming and people slipped away to sleep it off. All that remained of the party at dawn was a nutter and a psychiatrist's daughter still talking. We didn't sleep that night.

There were many sore heads the following morning; mine was not one of them. Despite the complete lack of sleep, the accumulation of exhaustion, and the alarming experience of the night before, I was remarkably upbeat. It was almost like being on a high and that was very unusual. The return journey held no fears any more. Even thoughts of going back to what passed for normality for me made no impact on my mood; that would only hit me later. I took a cab to the station as others struggled with their baggage. I was mildly surprised that a Mercedes picked us up; there seemed an odd style to that. I bought a final pack of *Gauloises*, sans filtres at the station; being linguistically challenged, smoking local cigarettes was always my way when abroad, my vague attempt at the culture of others. We made it to and across Paris without a hitch then boarded the *Eurostar* for home. Many slept but I was still on my alien high. At Ashford International we said our goodbyes and I headed back to my world.

I think it must have been a Friday the day we returned. That evening still in a personably unreal state I headed off along the road, down the hill and entered the little pub at the bottom. It was packed as ever for the start of the weekend. I bought a pint and headed over to look for the usual crowd. I spotted Emma sat by the open fire at the far end of the bar and joined her there in one of the armchairs. I expected a greeting of sorts but not the one I got.

"I've just had my nipple pierced, do you want to see it?" That really did take me aback. Being unsure how to respond to that in a crowded pub I declined. The freshly pierced nipple was flashed several times that night but it would be about three years before I actually got to see; such piercings were far less common then than they are now; strange how fashions change.

We drank for a couple of hours then moved on to another pub at the other end of town that had a late licence at weekends; almost the whole town congregated there when everywhere else shut. It was only then that the effects of not sleeping for forty eight hours finally struck. The others went off to watch the stripper at a particularly raucous stag do at the other end of the pub. I just sat there. The stag party ended in tears but I missed that bit; I had quietly slipped off home. Taking three of my blue and white capsules I went to bed with few thoughts of what the morrow would bring. I expected a long lie in then back to my usual despair.

It was the phone that woke me up. The sedative power of the pills was so great that I usually slept through noise. That morning I didn't. No one answered. I struggled out of bed very disorientated. I scrabbled around on the bedside table looking for my glasses then looked at my watch. It was 8 o'clock. Still the phone kept on. Inside I was furious. This had better be fucking good went the voice of my thoughts. It was still ringing as I stumbled down the stairs. Still in a state of confusion I lifted the receiver.

"Hello."

"Is that Tony?"

"No, it's Mark." I was seething.

"It's Father Michael, is your dad there?" Whilst I had utterly rejected religion, my parents were quite devout Christians. Indeed my father was church warden at their church. Despite my beliefs or lack of them Michael was a good man and a very good priest. For him to be calling at that time of the morning meant that it must be important.

"No, he's out."

"Can you get him to call me? There's been a fire at the church." In fact it had been fire bombed. It was a strange return to reality, and not one I needed on such little sleep.

Chapter 24

Potential

The *Right Illness Theory* states that the seriousness with which a patient is treated is directly proportional to the given diagnosis. Amongst those who call themselves professionals there always seemed to be a hierarchy of illness. At the top were schizophrenia and manic depression, near the bottom was depression, and right down, the lowest of the low, those deemed to have a Personality Disorder. Whatever the label that was chosen for me, I was positioned in the lowest echelons of mental illness. The slightly cynical and more frivolous extension to the theory was that the difference between those with manic depression and those with depression was that the former were usually trying to prove that they were not ill, and the latter that they were ill. The bottom line in mental illness was that those without a psychotic diagnosis had very little chance of being treated seriously. And those who were decreed to have a disordered personality were considered untreatable. The legacy of god and the Hotel still hung over me. As time passed my regrets at having agreed to go there grew.

Whilst it was a disaster to be put in the final box, the dustbin of mental health, there were also major disadvantages to being in the top ones. Those with psychotic diagnoses lived with two major fears: the side effects of the drugs; and being put in hospital either on a voluntary basis or under a section of the 1983 Mental Health Act. The response to these twin fears was twofold: people often didn't take their medication; and they didn't tell the shrinks the truth a lot of the time. This in itself extended the them and us scenario and the belief held by many of us that they were the enemy. I had always believed that I had a psychotic illness and had long since rejected the labels given to me. No one seemed prepared to accept that maybe there was another option. There was no objective challenge to their views particularly after god had spoken. I had often wondered why they hadn't at least tried the anti psychotic route. I had seen the word psychotic in my notes but it had never been mentioned to me in person.

By 1996 the world of psychosis was changing. There were new drugs on the market, the so called atypicals which in many cases were more effective with fewer side effects than their predecessors. Their advent had helped Matt to turn his life around. I'd known others too who had had major changes in their conditions because of atypicals, and without too many problems. I had talked to them as honestly as I could for some time but they appeared to dismiss my claims. Now, in the light of the *Zadok* incident, my life and my illness had changed. I was left with the dilemma of whether to tell the quiet, mild mannered man what had happened or to just leave it. To be taken more seriously though, to abide by the *Right Illness Theory*, I decided the best way forward was to tell it as it had happened and hope that the benefits would outweigh any possible negatives. Maybe, just maybe, they would accept my word and respond in an appropriate manner. Finally there was potential for change and progress.

With the unusual high of the end of the trip all too brief I returned to type as I waited to see the shrink. Things got worse in early August as they always did; another of my times. Time too was drifting on in another summer. For all the people and all the parties I was still me. The really bad times didn't seem to last quite so long now but they were just as intense as they had always been. Although my mind was made up to tell him what had happened I still had little faith that he would do anything. Why would this shrink be different? Pleasant though he was he had hardly been very proactive. He had twice increased my medication. He'd even offered me a week's "holiday" in hospital when I was really bad but it was hardly an attractive proposition. I had, of course, declined.

It was the middle of August when I saw him; just another summer's day at the usual place. I sat down as always and we got under way. I just talked and told him what had happened. As I spoke he looked more animated and worried than normal. Then he started to question me very closely. The longer it went on the more I began to think that maybe he was finally beginning to believe me. It seemed a much longer visit than normal. He appeared different. He really was beginning to believe. Then he asked me a last question.

"Do you get obsessive about things?"
"No, not really." With that he seemed to revert to type.

A Pillar of Impotence

I think it was on that day that they finally accepted that I did have a psychotic illness. It is hard to tell as I cannot read minds and I'd not looked at my notes since just after leaving the Hotel. Subsequent events did prove that at some stage it was accepted that I did indeed have a psychotic illness. That day in August I told my story, he listened, and maybe accepted. Accepted but did nothing. It would be another five years before the significance of missing this potential opportunity became clear. Life could have been so very different.

Whilst there was little joy from my dealings with the shrink, all was not lost. Jayne, the woman who had been so guarded when I had met her some eighteen months before had, over time, become more approachable. Now she proved to be an unlikely ally. She turned out to have a rare ability to listen to my troubles and show an understanding that seemed beyond the capabilities of those who had trained to do just that. As the summer began to wane into autumn we often talked on a real level. With others all around we could often be found shut off from them, deep in intense conversation. She, like James, became someone I could really talk to; I knew many people now but only those two really understood.

The end of the summer was a time of mixed emotions. The students moved off back to their respective places of study. This brought other opportunities which had not existed even two years before. My travels to Sussex became less frequent but now Portsmouth, Bristol, and Newcastle were within the sights of my itinerance. The first I would achieve on several occasions, the second would take some time to achieve whilst the third would always be in my intentions but never realised. The end of September brought a regular pair of concerts to do, then, with the students all gone, I settled back into the tedium of autumn. Nothing was on the horizon, I merely went back to trying to fight my way through each day hoping it would not be too bad. Life was but an existence, and a lonely one at that.

It was a Wednesday evening in early October. As was my habit I went down to the MIND centre, a chance to get together with my brethren, my companions in the shadows. There was nothing out of the ordinary going on that day, it was just another day. Whilst talking with Heather something unusual happened.

"I've got something that might interest you. There's a meeting next week at the Day Service about education for the mentally ill. Will you come along?"

"Why not?" That surprised me. I was very sceptical of education. In the early days they had said to me that I should go to college but I couldn't see the point. I had education coming out of every orifice and after Cambridge there seemed little to gain from going back in. And that was without even thinking about how ill I was. I could barely read a word let alone study. This was of course perceived as me not wanting to get better, another loaded choice.

I wondered for a long time after the conversation why I had agreed to go. How on earth could they help me? What would I learn that I didn't already know? Maybe I was just supporting our cause. And maybe I had nothing to lose. If there was the slightest chance that it would help I was willing to gamble. I'd tried everything else. As things stood I had Caroline, and whilst that helped in the very short term I couldn't see any dramatic progress, or indeed that the latter might come at all. Strangely it never occurred to me that it might provide the first stepping stone to going home, home to Cambridge; life was still hour by hour, day by day.

I still had the battered yellow VW with the cracked indicator light in the autumn of 1996. I'd lost track of the number of times I'd driven down the well worn route to the Day Service. It had been nearly five years since I'd first set foot in that place. There had been many false dawns in those five years; so many options but none had worked. The subterranean lift didn't seem to go up and down as often but it remained below ground level and would still slump at an alarming rate. Suicide was a constant companion, waiting to happen. As I drove over there one more time the prospective evening seemed just like so many others before; I'd try anything but held out little hope. It was just another flawed attempt at helping those who could not be helped.

When I arrived there were the usual familiar faces; those looking for something, anything that could end their misery. There were two unfamiliar faces, hovering around a table bedecked with leaflets, their backs turned to the windows that looked out over the fishing pond. It was a peaceful place where I often sat. They were both in their forties in my estimation, a man and a woman. She was short and blonde but lacked presence. He was bearded with a worldly look to him, a man who had seen much. Their dress came across a too formal for such an occasion, but they came from the real world, the one we all aspired to but were unable to reach.

They made an enthusiastic presentation to outline their proposition. It would be a course specifically and only for those with enduring mental health problems. It would by necessity be gently paced and designed initially to support students back into an educational environment. Many in the past had tried the education route but most had failed at the first sign of relapse. Now there would be support before and when people were ready to move into the mainstream. It seemed a plausible idea but whether it would work was open to question; it is easy to give the hard sell, the promises made, but far more difficult to convert the potential. I wasn't really sure what to make of it when they were speaking but I had been struck by the apparent confidence of the bearded man.

With the formalities over I took the chance to speak to him over coffee. It quickly became clear that he was not only confident he could make it work but also that he truly believed in what he was doing. He also gave off a strong sense that he genuinely cared for us and about what he wanted to do. He was, quite simply, plausible. I left in the little yellow car only partially convinced by the evening's events. It was the man who had been convincing more than the concept, but I still had my usual scepticism in my mind. I needed clarification on the bearded man, the man we would simply know as Ian. There were certain advantages to living next door to the Vice Principal of the college, and gathering information was one of them.

The next time I saw my neighbour I asked him about this man, this Ian. "Good bloke" was the response. That was enough to make me agree despite my doubts. It would prove to be a very significant night; ultimately it would match the chance meeting with Caroline. I didn't realise it but another major part of the puzzle had just fallen into place; the seed had been sown but it would need time to germinate and that time would not even start until after Easter. In the mean time there was yet another Christmas to get through and that meant the lift slumping to the floor; such was my life in mid winter.

It was in the run up to Christmas that I made my monthly pilgrimage to see the quiet shrink. Nothing had happened since the *Zadok* incident, we had just been over the same things and the same questions that characterised our meetings. He'd been quite intrigued by what I was doing with Caroline and, unlike his predecessors, had not challenged my trying my own way. In fact he accepted that it was of benefit if only for a short time. But he himself had done nothing new, we were simply maintaining the status quo. I wasn't expecting anything out of the ordinary but this day it would be different. It all started as usual; then he surprised me.

"I know you are having some periods of relative stability but I also realise you are still very unhappy." That's an understatement. "Would you consider doing some more Psychotherapy?" The immediate, painful, and futile thoughts of the past flashed back to me. My previous experiences had been negative, and, in the case of the Hotel, tinged with regret. But I was desperate. Like the idea of the college I was prepared to do anything.

"Would it be with you?" That may have seemed like an odd question to him but it had been done by a shrink before. I could visualise being able to handle it with him but I wasn't sure about another stranger.

"No, I was thinking of referring you to the Psychotherapy department. There's probably a long waiting list so you might have to wait some time."

"I suppose it's worth a go, why not?" With that the die was cast.

Only time would tell if any of these options might make a difference. I didn't have much faith, but then again, what little faith I had ever had had long been dissipated by repeated failures. But like the ultimatum at the Hotel, what choice did I have? For now it was just time to wait.

Chapter 25

Life's Waiting Room

For many of us reality was an alarming prospect. What was there for us in the real world? What did being well really mean? How would we know when we were well? These were some of the questions that vexed us. Whilst people often talked about the relatively large percentage of the population who would at some point have mental health problems, there is a much smaller proportion of those people who would have long term illnesses. We were the ones who didn't respond to treatment, or those for whom treatment only offered a kind of holding operation. In that respect we were different. The longer one suffers the harder it is to remember exactly what real life is like. To me normal meant not being mentally ill any more. Much as I desired to get well I couldn't see what awaited me when I got to the promised land. There were of course pressures on all of us from the real world. Much of the Mental Health System seemed dedicated to getting its patients or clients as they often called us out the door and back into work as fast as possible. Then there was the age old enemy, the DSS as they were now known. As far as they were concerned the more people they could get off the books the better. What they failed to see was just how tough it was to get work even if one became well enough so to do. Economists talk of the poverty trap; we were well and truly living in it. Stigma did not only exist in the barbers.

Yet by mid winter, as I waited for so many things, I had already taken a tentative first step into reality. Once a week, for a couple of hours, I had started to help children to learn to read. I actually rather liked it. The kids liked it, their teachers appreciated it, but above all there was no pressure. They were aware of my situation and just accepted it. The biggest problem for me was the early hour. Yet each week during term time, I set off with my mum to give my time. Time was an entity I possessed in abundance. School was one of the very few things in my life that had any meaning. As was the way in my world, it had to be a secret. Any hint of being able to do anything and the DSS would start their hounding.

They were, of course, already hounding me on another front. It had been two and a half years since the fight for DLA had started. There was still no news as to when I would be going to the second tribunal. That was very much a mixed situation. I had missed out on so many opportunities because they had opposed me from the start but at least I didn't have the worry and stress of the tribunal coming up. The original low level award had been made for a period of three years. As was their procedure, they sent out renewal forms six month before the expiry date. So it was that in February 1997 yet another brown A4 envelope made its way through my letterbox from them. It was time to start all over again. With Heather's help the now familiar booklets were completed and sent off. A few weeks later another brown envelope arrived. The result was the same. Back to waiting.

As I settled back into what passed for a routine in my life there was a subtle shift. It had been two and a half years since the DLA application. But it had also been a similar length of time since I left the Hotel, and, by extension, since I had been smoking regularly. It had been a lifeline in that time. I was certain that had I not started when I did, I would by now have succumbed to the desperate craving for death and the release that that seemed to offer. There had been many changes in that time but the bottom line was that the fundamentals had not shifted. I was still in pain and there was only one way out in my mind. Hash had regularly halted those feelings but they were usually there again in the morning. It was simply something that I needed. It had a grip but for the most part it was a good grip, one more potent and effective than any of the many pills I had taken. I had a need for the blue and white capsules but only to affect the need for sleep that was such a constant factor in my madness. I had woven an intricate web for survival, one that was dependent on foreign substances both natural and synthetic, and on those within my circle. This was the scaffold on which I teetered. The loss of one constituent could so easily push me into pulling the lever to the trap door. Life and existence were precarious despite my waiting. To venture into unknown territory was indeed a gamble; to take that risk was fraught with danger and fear.

With change or the potential for change that faced me in the first quarter of the year a ripple effect happened. The strained strand of the web proved to be the hash. It started to go bad on me as I journeyed back each night. It started slowly with just a few nights of starting to think. Thinking had always been my downfall in the illness. It just got out of control. Hash had always halted this for me. Now it began to encourage it. The more I thought the less I slept. The less I slept the more I got ill. The more I got ill the more I thought. And it was the thought of reality, whatever that may be, that fuelled the process. It became unpleasant to smoke but I couldn't stop. It was now part of me as much as my pills, and it was beginning to control me, not me it.

Changes in the air were not just confined to my small portion of the world. In the wider scheme of things the end of an era was coming. I had very clear memories of the political world that had been the mid to late 70s despite my young age. It had been eighteen years since Thatcher came to power. She in turn had been gone for almost eight years. The remnants of a lengthy Tory administration were wavering on the brink of calamity as winter turned to spring. Electioneering was in full swing and the once obscure political figure was no longer so obscure. With the election coming the old nemesis of so many British governments reappeared with great cunning and style. As the main political parties campaigned so did the IRA. It was against this backdrop that my life took another very unexpected turn.

My father had retired in the same year as the last election. He still worked part time but it had given them an opportunity to do other things. My mum had finally managed to realise her dream of flying on Concorde amongst other travels. Such times had little effect on me. I merely went off to see Miriam for a few days and enjoyed the relative peace. Travelling for me was limited to visiting friends and the occasional choir trip. It had been right at the start that I had last actually been on a holiday where I didn't have to sing. France in 1990 still held an immense and painful resonance for me despite the seven years that had passed since. Nothing was on the cards that spring.

It was a quite unusual and often uncomfortable occasion to go out to eat with my parents. There was however a rather nice pub nearby called the Marquis of Granby that they rather liked. It must have been in late March or early April that I found myself in the car with them headed out for lunch. Other than the fact we were actually going out to eat there was nothing unusual about the day. The restaurant was renowned for its fish dishes. One of the more bizarre experiences of my illness was that I had developed an aversion to fish; too little appetite, too many bones, don't want to eat. I avoided the fish and, part way through some meat dish or other the conversation from my dad changed and he took me completely by surprise.

"We've been checking the finances and we think we can take you to Jordan on Concorde." What? Going to Petra had long been my dream. "It's a bit too hot for mum but you could go with me or one of your friends." They can't be serious. But they were. What do they want? Why? Why now? As so often happened when I was surprised my mind went overboard. I was quite literally stunned and became very unsteady on the small bar stool on which I perched. What do I do? Do I accept? I can't accept, it's too much. Confusion. The exhilaration was tempered by a feeling of suspicion. I had had so little from them in the past but an education. Now they were offering something beyond value to me. My mind thought about what they wanted in return. There had to be strings attached but they weren't obvious. As ever I hedged my bets.

"I'll think about it." Then lunch continued as if nothing had happened. My mind careered on on the same path.

I accepted a couple of days later with many doubts. The trip was due in October. A long way to go and yet more to ponder as I waited.

As the final days and weeks of the old political order waned so the campaign from across the rough western seas had a greater effect on our everyday lives. As a small child I could vividly remember being evacuated from a military open day due to a bomb threat. That was the early 70s. We had moved in 1974 and the first time my parents phoned their old priest from the new house he was recovering from cradling the dying at the site of the Guildford pub bombing; they had known nothing of the carnage until making that call. But it always seemed to be something that happened to others. That changed the day I watched the news and saw a familiar phone box in London. It was outside one of my haunts on the edge of China Town. A bomb had been planted inside then a warning sent. Once again mortality stared me in the face. It was another of those curious twists of fate and chance that kept me in Kent that day. The following year I would come much closer to a bomb very nearby.

The campaign did however catch up with me shortly after. I spent a few days with Miriam in April. It had been some years since the train operators had changed their ticketing system to my detriment. In the early years of my madness I had regularly spent a week or two at the time in Sussex or elsewhere. Then they made returns valid for only five days. More costs and disruption. It was on the final day of my ticket's validity when the campaign affected me. Bomb warnings paralysed the rail network in and out of London. I was stuck. Whilst it was better being there it looked as if it would be an expensive inconvenience. With good grace the ticket was honoured and I returned the next day. It just seemed so easy to do. Yet the election campaign ground on regardless; we were all still British of course and the Dunkirk spirit held sway at such times of crisis.

On 1st May the Tories were swept from power by the New Labour landslide. Change had finally come and the images of the once obscure one were everywhere. Perhaps more telling were the pictures of his wife the following day as flowers were delivered to Number 10. Neither would I forget Gerald Kaufmann's speech at the start of the new parliament and his reference to the "the iron heal of the Minister without Portfolio." Blair did not come alone and new meaning for an old word would enter our everyday language. The age of the institutionalised spin doctor had arrived. Spin or no spin New Labour enjoyed a remarkably long honeymoon period in the months that followed. Our world had changed in some ways but not in others. The question of how different New Labour was to the Tories would become a common topic of conversation amongst those who cared. For those who didn't, it was end of an era they knew as Thatcherism and all the pain that that had brought to too many. It was not a view shared by most from my past.

May also heralded the start of the new venture at the college. The seeds had been sown the previous October, and now, as the weather warmed, the first germination of a new scheme emerged from the uneven and stony ground that underpinned the lives of a small group of mentally ill people residing on the East Kent coast. It was all very gentle. We met once a week for a couple of hours late in the day. It was quieter then. We all knew each other before hand which just left Ian and his assistant to get to know us. I still had many doubts about what if anything I could learn but it was only a small gamble. What he did have to offer though was an introduction to an area that terrified me; that bane of modern life and work, the computer. As the first couple of weeks went by I quickly realised that what I had to learn came from the man himself. More importantly though, he was learning from us. He was stepping into our world as much as we were stepping into his. Two apparently disparate worlds were colliding; the chaos of the mad with the discipline of education. But he just seemed to make it work. For the first time in many years I was confronted by intellectual conversation on a regular basis.

I'd only been there a couple of weeks when I received a rather unexpected phone call. Over the years I'd more or less lost touch with the old Cambridge crowd. A few had come to the Hotel to visit me but since then almost nothing. One friend had called out of the blue one evening in that time; he wanted to know why his brother had tried to commit suicide and I was the logical choice to attempt an answer to such a vexing question. I still held my fear of phones even though calls had been a lot more numerous recently. I was rather surprised when a call came up the stairs to say that an old housemate was on the phone. The surprise was heightened when he invited me to a Bumps party in Cambridge. I was surprised but also frightened; it was at that time of year and at the same event that it had started in the all too clear but distant past. Fear or not I accepted straight away. Maybe I would cope better now, especially if I could induce the haze that had been my almost constant companion for nearly three years.

The weeks slipped by quickly to the party. As expected I was ill but the face of my public persona was well versed. The memories and flashbacks haunted me that weekend but were tempered by finally re-establishing relations with the few who had known me before. They were accepting and pleased to see me but still struggling with how to react to me. The smoke helped though. For one night only it was back to old times. Some of my memories at least were happy ones. What was most interesting was that they were the ones likely to lose out in the political shift that had just happened but they were not bothered. In a limited way I was back in the fold. Only time would tell if I would remain there. Slowly and almost innocuously another piece of the puzzle dropped into place. What I could not see then was the bigger picture. Elements of change were there early that summer but they were still very disjointed in my mind.

It was shortly after a generally pleasant weekend in my true home that another of the elements made its first tentative appearance. I had been waiting for seven months when the appointment came through. My next venture into the world of Psychotherapy began on a stifling day in July. I travelled to Ashford with my normal confused mind, tinged again with a healthy dose of cynicism. I had few expectations but, as had been the case from the start, I was willing to try anything. The first meeting was a pleasant surprise. She was very good at making me feel at ease and I talked with few qualms. The following week we met again with much the same result. I was beginning to think that maybe I had found someone who I might be able to trust. It must have been on about the third visit that she dropped a bombshell. It had started as before with the same ease of conversation. Nothing was out of the ordinary, then the dramatic change.

"I want you to join a group that I'm starting up in September."
"No way am I doing group therapy again." I didn't even think about that one but memories of the Hotel immediately deluged my conscious mind.
"Well, if you want to do individual work you'll have to wait at least another seven months and I can't guarantee it will be with me."

There I was cornered again. No one had even mentioned the possibility of doing group work before. There was a choice but it was a loaded one. With great reluctance I agreed deciding that it had been far too long in the waiting already and another seven months was too much more time. As I drove home the old doubts took over. There was also a feeling of having been deceived. Yet as with the ultimatum at the Hotel was there a choice?

We had a break from the college over the summer. It had been an initial foray into the unknown but one that felt safe. The real test would be in September. The upcoming start of autumn held the prospect of much change. Jordan was that bit closer, a group of new people awaited me in a once familiar setting, and the college would be that much more real. In the meantime though there was the rest of the summer party season to negotiate.

It had been two years since the epic summer of '95 and change had come to all of us. The people were the same yet their lives were slowly but surely moving on. They changed jobs, they changed relationships and they moved from being students to something more real. With it came subtle changes in our relationships with each other. The pub at the bottom of the hill was still lively but not as often as it had been. New faces appeared but there were fewer and fewer of them. The insignificant seaside town itself was caught up in the shift. Cracks were appearing in what had been familiar, and familiar was safe. But the cracks were almost imperceivable at times. The weekend was still the weekend and the intentions of us all had changed little. There were still parties to go to and one would be yet another birthday as time marched on to thirty.

It was well into August when I had my final one to one meeting with the woman in Ashford. We were but a couple of weeks from the proposed start of the forthcoming group yet I had no idea where it would be held.

"Where will the group be held?" I asked in all innocence.
"I've told you that but you've blotted it out." What the fuck does that mean? I was mystified by such an obtuse answer.
"You haven't told me."
"Yes I have."
"If you did I don't remember."
"It's at Western Avenue."
"Where's that? I've never heard of it." She looked embarrassed and paused for a second, apparently not sure what to say.
"I'm sorry I thought I'd told you and you'd blotted it out because it is a Day Service." Bollocks. What bullshit. My mind erupted in fury and contempt. We'd not even started and her own stupidity and delusion had seriously undermined any belief I had in her. What difference was there between her and the rest? Furious though I was I let it slip by. It was but another fuck up by a professional and I was very used to those by then.

A Pillar of Impotence

My birthday fell on a Saturday that year. A good day for a birthday. I'd been to a birthday barbecue the previous Saturday so it had been a good week for seeing people. On that Saturday at the end of August, a time I'd so hated when growing up, I headed down the hill to the little pub quite early. There were many friends there, some by invitation, others out of habit. We were all drunk at closing time and wondering where to go next. One of the company was house sitting for a relative that weekend and invited us back. The party went on long into the night as was our norm. We were oblivious to the rest of the world and most of the rest of the world, the neighbours excepted, were oblivious to us.

As we drank and smoked, a couple left the Ritz in Paris and got into a waiting Mercedes. They drove off into the night hotly pursued by the press. The car crashed in a Paris underpass. The couple died sending shock waves around the world. The first I knew of it was about 9.30 the next morning. I wasn't happy to be woken at such an early hour by my mother. She uttered one sentence.

"Princess Diana's been killed in a car crash." Some wake up call.

Chapter 26

Og the King of Basan

My exposure to the Bible started very young. We were regular church goers and I loved the stories that were told. As I didn't learn to read until I was eight years old they remained as stories until I went away to school; then they became day to day occurrences. Much of what we sang was Biblically based so we sang the services and the responses, listened to sung prayers and intoned the strange words of the psalms every day. I didn't realise it then but I had been right about the stories in my childhood for that was what they were: tales from long ago about characters and events that had a basis in fact but no one is certain exactly what happened. And from those stories came three of the great Monotheistic religions of the world; the same stories up to a point but different beliefs and outcomes. What ties it all together is this thing people call God. Even as a child he seemed a very contradictory figure, vengeful in one moment, soothing and forgiving in the next epitomised best in the words of the psalms. Some days they were tedious and long, others they were short and triumphant. We all dreaded the 15th evening of the month for that brought us the infamous Psalm 78; it was long yet extraordinary in its diversity and illustration of the two sides of the Deity. Then I hated it, today I listen to it. But it was another character from the psalms who always made us laugh and smile, the splendidly named Og the King of Basan. Like so many others he was slain by the Israelites to avenge their God.

It was like that with the man who conducted us. Ostensibly we were there to enhance the worship of that very same God. People came from all over the world to that chapel either for worship or just to hear us. That was the public persona. However, no one was allowed to watch us rehearse. In the morning the room was our room. In the afternoons, or on Sunday mornings that place of worship was closed to the public. There were moments of great triumph, euphoria and pleasure to go along with a modicum of boredom. He was a great motivator but the moments of retribution were prolonged and savage. I'd first been exposed to them on the very first day when an eleven year old was late. But it was our secret. There was the public face and the private one, and the two never met. Maybe that was why rehearsal was closed although that never occurred to us at the time. He never hit the adults in that place of worship, only us. But they weren't exempt; humiliation was just another form of abuse and reinforcement. The message had to be reinforced all the time. We must be the best in the world. It left a legacy for so many of us, but that too was our secret. The world within a world, the public and the private. It was never talked about, it just was.

In my late twenties I sometimes thought about those days. Then I would get angry. I would turn the anger in on myself. The music would start in my head. That was usually followed by the voices. Control was lost. On rare occasions the mental jukebox would play those very same psalms. It was never the joyful and triumphant ones that echoed in my mind, always the dark and dangerous ones in the minor keys. They were the ones that were accusatory: you have sinned and need to be punished. With that condemnation the questions came. Why? What have I done? What the fuck have I done to deserve this? They were thoughts, but they were no less under my power to stop than the music or the voices themselves. I would sit for hours listening and thinking but there was never an answer. So many of us asked that question; the why me? But we never came up with an answer, just the vague thought we must have done something terrible and deserved the pain. In September 1997 those thoughts were not uppermost in my mind. There was a great deal of change coming in the next couple of months. Change was frightening but I was trying as hard as I could to face it. Og and his compatriots were nowhere to be seen.

Early autumn saw me take two separate steps, one into reality, and one further into unreality. It just worked out that both fell on a Tuesday. The college was a rather more frenetic place than it had seemed during those late afternoons in the summer. We were all familiar, as were the surroundings, it was just those who adorned our surroundings that had changed. There were people everywhere most of whom seemed to be lost. In their midst was that small group who were lost in a different way. Crowds still worried me so it was something of fight just to stay there but stay I did. The first couple of weeks we had to deal with a certain amount of bureaucracy but that was the norm for us; the DSS had long honed us into that path. Bewildering though the pace of life had become, it was still gentle in the classroom. Not much to learn initially except the machines that I had come to loath but accept as part of my future, whatever that might bring. But there was a very early hint of a scarier prospect for me. He mentioned almost in passing that he wanted for us to try to make a presentation on something of interest and then write about it. Since the days of the Palace, writing had become one of my greatest fears; that meant being judged, again.

Whilst I took those tentative steps towards reality in the day, by night I ventured back into the dark recesses of unreality. I had many reservations about going back into to group therapy but little choice. So in the still light of the early September evenings I drove my battered yellow VW north west on the route to London. A few miles up the road I turned off to Ashford and the next step along the conventional route to well being. We sat in a warm room on soft but noisy chairs warily eyeing those around us and wondering what we were each there for. It was not new to me but it became clear very quickly that it was to the others. Unlike the usual experience of the Hotel the silence was broken very quickly in the first session. The inquisitive one was the first to speak. Then slowly each of us spoke and the start of what was always going to be a complex scenario began to emerge. My first impressions were that I quite liked the others. There was none of the hostility of my previous experiences but it was made easier by the fact that we all started at the same point. There were prior dramas and tales to deal with, but it was a blank canvas ready to be developed by us. There was, however, something that seemed to be out of place, I just couldn't work out what it was.

Those first weeks of September saw change for me but it was relatively comfortable. But an interruption was about to take place. Even in those few short weeks of autumn I developed a sense of guilt about letting them all down because of the interlude but it was too important. The trip to Jordan started on 1st October, and, guilt or no guilt that was in my path now.

The last night of September was spent in an expensive but dreary hotel at Heathrow Airport. For the first time since we'd moved to Kent when I was nine I was to spend time alone with my dad. After dinner I adjourned to the bar to watch Liverpool and Celtic and to lose myself in my own thoughts. It was a strangely anxious night full of worry and expectation. I'd looked forward for so long in a time where there was rarely much to look forward to yet I was nervous. Fear of exhaustion, of the unknown, of the guilt, and perhaps foremost in my mind the fear of the strangers with whom I would travel. Whilst we lived in the same house, my dad did not live in my world and I had worked so hard to keep them both out of there. Three strangers under one roof passing and conversing in an obtuse way. My world was my world and only those from that world were let in. I knew nothing of him, nor he of me. Then there were the others I would meet in the morning. Would I be honest? Would they accept me? Would they humour me? Would they like me? These thoughts crowded my mind as sat alone in a quiet bar. The night proved to be tense and, for most part, sleepless. Then came the early check in.

I was shattered the next morning. There were formalities to get through and although handled with a great deal of style as befits a Concorde trip the first part of the day did little to lift my mood. When we boarded I still felt like crashing out but knew there was no way I could or would. Even the question "would you like champagne?" made no impact. I was tired and nervous. We taxied out at a gentle pace with few thoughts of what the next few minutes would be like. Then it happened. The afterburners kicked in, the brakes came off and we thundered down the Heathrow tarmac, pinned to our seats at a speed few could imagine. As the flames spewed from the four huge engines the adrenaline fired through my veins and took me in an instant to a different place. There was no tiredness left just an incredible buzz.

Lunch took three hours at an altitude so high the sky was black above us. Then came the choice, port or cognac? The port was most welcome although I missed the opportunity for a fine cigar with it. But in that atmosphere it mattered not a jot. Here was a world of great privilege, one that I knew would come but once in my lifetime. Time stood still up there. In only three hours or so it was over. We disembarked to the forty degree heat of Aqaba and a warm Arab welcome. It was just the start. Even the coach journey seemed so different to the many I had undertaken before. The world was different again on the ground. When we finally arrived at the hotel high up in the mountains close to Petra most were exhausted for a second time. More was to come though with an evening feast planned.

Early in the evening I found myself alone wandering around the complex in its breathtaking surroundings. I was tired again, the adrenaline having burned itself out. Then I discovered the Turkish Bath. Intrigued I walked in, paid my money and headed to the steam room. In the stifling atmosphere I reflected on what had already been a long day and what was to come. It felt as if I would dissolve in there leaving only a neat pile of bones. Time elongated in the heat just as it did in the land of the mad. Eventually I was led out for an extraordinary massage. As I sat after wrapped from head to foot in towels, sipping sweet tea I was overtaken by a sense of feeling completely reborn. I had experienced nothing like it in my travels and knew I would have to go back again.

The feast went remarkably well despite the extremely cold temperature of the mountain night. My fears of meeting others and their reaction to me proved unfounded. I was considerably younger than almost anyone there yet they were all friendly. And my dad was just different, himself and carefree. The after effects of such a long day kicked in relatively quickly and I once again found myself alone and wandering. So much to think of but not of sleep just yet for I knew that would not come for a while. Just as the first vestiges of loneliness filtered into my conscious I heard the faint sound of an old and slightly out of tune piano playing. I headed for the sounds and gingerly walked through the door. Inside were all the tour people and one of the women I had met early in the morning. The drink was flowing and I was back in my element, the ground most familiar. It was late in the night when we all left and silently prepared for the morrow. I had survived a gruelling day. And on that morrow Petra awaited us.

It proved to be a typically glorious Middle Eastern morning, sun blazing in the sky but without the oppressive atmosphere I'd come to know in the Far East. Forewarned about the local exchange rate I approached Petra perched precariously on the back of a shy dappled horse. Going right through on horse back was no longer an option but at the slow pace with which I was just about comfortable, I marvelled at the rugged mountains before dismounting at the entrance to the Siq. My mind was unusually peaceful. We were guided through the Siq by the admirable Gus, a man we'd met on arrival. There was a vast throng going through but they mattered not to me. Then we took that final step from gloom into mesmerising light. I'd seen it on film as had so many others but nothing could possibly prepare any of us for that moment of splendid clarity. I walked back and forward for some time just trying to take it all in. Even of column of marching Germans could not detract from the majesty of that place. A few steps more and the world opened up from the rocks to the imposing edifice that is the Treasury. And with that came the hawkers and peddlers. They did their worse but made no impact. I was finally out of the shell that enclosed my mind.

There was of course so much more. It was simply vast. We stayed but a few hours in that ancient place, sometimes with Gus and sometimes alone. It was hard to tell whether his stories were true or not but he added to the day. I wandered in a place I'd dreamed of for so long, and, as I did so a change occurred. The peace of the coming stayed. There were no voices. Neither were there thoughts of death. I felt no guilt yet I'd taken no drug or drink. It had all stopped. In those few hours freedom came over me. The past was no longer controlling my mind. I'd only ever achieved that through foreign substances prescribed or bought. And the fear of the return of chaos was gone. I was at peace with myself without a feeling of it being but a truce in the war. The war had gone.

Peace remained throughout a day that took us into the desert with the Bedouin, back to the Turkish Bath and to another feast. Spirits were high amongst a friendly crowd as we ate, drank, and marvelled at the stamina of the belly dancer. As I'd done the previous night I retired to the small bar as most adjourned to bed. Over a Hookah pipe we all reflected on the day yet none realised just what a day it had been for me. In the early hours I looked out over the mountains alone. Even in my loneliness there was silence in my mind.

We flew to Amman the following afternoon and the calm still reigned. It was a calm in one way yet an extraordinary high in another. For the first time in seven years the subterranean lift had broken the surface. Even hungover and tired most of the pain had gone. I still had an intense headache but my mind had long since learned to adjust to that. What mattered was that the mental gymnastics had stopped. We arrived at another five star hotel late in the afternoon to find ancient episodes of *Neighbours* dubbed into Arabic on the TV. My father went for a swim and I made for the bar. It was then that the crash happened.

For two hours I sat alone with my thoughts and voices. Time stood still and those who passed me were but fleeting ghosts drifting in and out of my world. The urge to run swept over me but here there was nowhere to run to. I had none of the thoughts of a foreign nuthouse that had accompanied me in Chartres but I was aware that here it was infinitely more precarious. I dreaded seeing any of the party but I knew I had to face them later. There was no cannabis to stop the voices and urges. I was completely alone. Some of those I had met knew of my illness but none could do anything about it. Neither would I let anyone into my private world. Desolation obliterated the highs of the previous two days. Slowly I became aware of time and headed off to prepare for another night of revelry. As I dressed for dinner back came the mask, my other well versed clothing. Through that evening none noticed the turmoil, and as the alcohol flowed the pain became anaesthetised and disappeared. It was another very late one in a bar with a Welshman who was a friend of a friend. Even out there the world was a very small place. As we sat in that bar the lift broke through the surface again and the buzz returned. In the morning, with the anaesthetic worn off, it was mercifully still in the daylight.

In the coming days we kept up the relentless pace and splendour. We travelled considerably by day and feasted by night. It was on one such trip that the bus stopped amid yet more astonishing scenery. As usual we piled off to hear another of Gus's commentaries. This day I never made it passed his opening sentence.

"This is Basan." For a second I failed to recognise the name. Basan, that sounds familiar, my mind thinking in words as was my habit. Where did I hear that name? Basan. But it sounded like Bashan. Bashan. Basan. Og! There I was standing in the land of Og slain by the Israelites in the quiet recesses of ancient history. That suddenly made it all feel more real. Jordan was Jordan to me, not, as Rachel later described it, the Holy Land. A place that had been an obscure if occasionally uplifting one in my childhood. That evening as I spoke to a retired priest who pieced together another piece of the puzzle.

"Fat bulls of Basan close me in on every side" he said. Another of the psalms. I was very struck by what he had said for it seemed to just encapsulate the world of mental illness. And that stayed with me for many years; it was a phrase that would come in handy with another professional I had yet to meet.

We saw so many sites and sights, each meticulously and eloquently presented. The sun setting over the Dead Sea accompanied by Hookah pipes. Jerash. The delights of Amman itself. We lunched at an old Turkish fort out in the desert after travelling on the rail road destroyed by T.E. Lawrence and his followers. The Seven Pillars of Wisdom. It was all the stuff of fantasy and dream. And throughout it all my mind stayed still. She was quiet, the jukebox switched off, and thoughts of death banished from my conscious.

The final night brought us another extravagant dinner, a fat cigar, and a late one in the bar with the Concorde crew. We crossed the Mediterranean in eighty six minutes on our return and were struck by lightening coming into land. It was over.

I made it for last orders at the bottom of the hill on a warm Monday night in October. I left to soft rain and no spliff; tonight there was no need.

My world had changed ever so slightly. For the first time I had enjoyed myself yet felt no guilt. I had survived a week without weed and, with that, was able to break the hold it had on me. No more would it control me. The lift was still above the surface. Whilst I knew it would inevitably crash below again I could at least remember what it was like to live again. Jordan was the instigator of a small but significant loosening of the shackles of despair. That was very much needed in the first week of October 1997. The second week brought me to the last judgement. The battle with the DSS was about to be resolved one way or another. Fraud or disabled? My life was once again in the hands of those who knew me not and who had their own agenda.

Chapter 27

To Judge the Quick and the Dead

Death has a habit of uniting people, at least temporarily. The shockwaves sent by the death of Diana Princess of Wales engulfed the country, and, judging from comments made to me in Jordan, much of the rest of the world too. Lost in the grief to an extent was the death within days of Mother Theresa of Calcutta. Only history will tell which was the more significant. But the unity created by that crash was palpable for many weeks after the event. I'd never met Princess Diana but sudden death was something familiar to me. At twenty eight I had lost count of the number of friends and acquaintances taken at too young an age. Since I had been ill I'd lost three friends to suicide, others too from natural causes or accidents. By no means had I been to all their funerals but I had been to enough to see that the judgements of life count for little in death. It is always the good that people talk about and rarely the truth because it's often too unpalatable on such occasions. Those who had chastised the Princess in life were curiously silent in her death. Later of course there would be critics of both these famous people. Yet post death criticisms and judgements are so different to those heaped upon us whilst we live; in death we leave a legacy, in life we must just face the judgement.

In my world early death was perceived as an accepted face of madness. So many of us stared death down each and every day. We also had to stare down judgement and stigma. Perhaps the most feared judge of our lives was the institution we knew simply as the DSS. It had such power and influence over our lives that it was one of the most formidable adversaries in our world. To some it was life and death. I often mused on how many had been lost to suicide because of the actions of the faceless bureaucrats who put into action a deeply flawed system. For six years I had battled them as they seemingly opposed me every step of the way. Many times they had exacerbated my condition and driven me closer to the end. Now I had to face my final judgement.

By the time of my second tribunal Sally, who had so brilliantly yet unsuccessfully represented me before, had left for another job. She had been replaced by a quiet and slightly less charismatic colleague called Adam. Despite his completely different demeanour he came across as highly efficient and knowledgeable when dealing with such matters. The crux remained the same as it had been before, namely that due to the intense suicidal urges I suffered, urges greatly exacerbated by being alone, necessitated that I have someone around almost all the time. This was precisely the criteria for the level of benefit we sought. It had always seemed ironic and unjust that so many I knew got it despite living alone yet it was refused in my case even though I lived with my parents precisely because it was too risky to be alone. It was only on very rare occasions that I was alone, and those occasions when I was alone, usually when I was travelling, it was only for a few hours. When my parents were away I was always away too, either with Miriam or friends. The first time this had been flatly rejected on the grounds that there was "no evidence." Suicidal intent is by its very nature almost impossible to prove. It was still very vivid in my mind, that image of a shocked Sally simply shaking her head. Now it was down to Adam to prove what Sally could not do, however eloquently she had presented the case.

For reasons that were never explained I had to travel all the way to Maidstone for the second hearing. Adam joined me at Ashford and spent the journey perusing the notes. He was confident, I was not. I had no faith or trust in them, seeing them, as so many of us did as the enemy. None of us really believed they were impartial, my self more than most considering my past dealings with them. Anxiety grew as each mile of track disappeared from sight. By the time we got there I was physically shaking, and that was compounded by a gnawing feeling of nausea.

Time went haywire there. As we waited, time speeded up and became impossible to keep a track of. We were called into a very formally set out room with a large table separating us from the judges. Again there were three of them, a chairman, a doctor, and a representative from the voluntary sector. Before me sat a substantial jug of water and two glasses. My first reaction was to pour a drink and sip nervously. This would continue throughout. Time almost stood still now. The chairman, perhaps wary of the lack of explanation given by the last tribunal, was very careful and precise as he introduced the panel and set out the procedures to follow. He was very different to his predecessor, more deliberate and in control. Then the questions started. Some I fielded, others were left to Adam. Even when speaking though I felt a curious detachment from the events unfolding before me. It was another intensely unnerving experience. On and on the questions came at us, and all the time I sipped, sweated, and became more uncomfortable. The doctor seemed very dubious about me but the expected attack that had been launched by his medical colleague never happened. When it was over we were sent out to await my fate. Relieved as I was to be away from the questioning, the nerves were still frayed as we waited. Time was still running slowly but it was hard to know what to make of that. Adam was just as confident as he had been before going in; I was expecting the worst.

We were called back in after another indeterminate period of time. Back to the water. But an expected yes or no answer failed to materialise. He went into a slow and precise explanation of their findings, mindful as ever of possible recrimination and come back. Finally he told us that the appeal had been upheld by a majority of two to one. Once again though, the doctor had voted against me. That took some of the impact of the success away but for the first time that day some form of calm returned to my demeanour. I was handed some paper work to sign. At the bottom, where the dates for the award were listed, his hand writing was a little unclear: the 4 of 1994 was difficult to decipher and he had left a 0 off 2000. Thinking nothing of it I said nothing, signed, and handed them back. After four years of fighting it was over.

I was in a much better and calmer mood as we headed south east on the train. Just as Adam got off at Ashford he gave me some parting words.

"It should take about six weeks before the money comes through. If you haven't heard by early December give me a ring." With that he was gone. It was hard to get over the sense of triumph tinged with relief as I sat alone for the short distance to the coast. I had waited too long and missed so many opportunities. Now with the back dated giro some of my life would be so much easier. For all of that though I was still ill, and, at its worst money made no difference. I knew that those times would come to me again but for now there was something to celebrate.

A Pillar of Impotence

The weeks that followed seemed to pass very quickly. Fresh from the events in Maidstone my mood was quite upbeat. The darkness of autumn and winter had always had the opposite effect on me; whilst most became increasingly depressed over the months of the long nights and short, cold, damp days, I found the dark and dreary hours easier to deal with than the heat and light of summer. I settled into my new routine as best I could.

At the college Ian was as good as his word. I spent a short part of my morning talking about Jordan using photographic illustrations. Then, for the first time in six years started to do some research. I was slower than I'd once been but had not really lost my ability to do it. I feared the writing process that would follow but I had developed an unusual enthusiasm and determination to achieve some sort of result which outweighed the inevitable judgement of the conclusion. In the afternoons I fought on with the computers with rather less enthusiasm and much more stress. On the whole though, the first parts of Tuesdays were okay. The evenings brought group therapy; that was rather less happy.

Throughout the autumn and early winter I spent an hour and a half each week sitting on less than comfortable chairs, listening and talking to a seemingly disparate collection of people. We were still feeling each other out, many often talking in riddles, not in the abrupt and blunt manner that had regularly characterised my stay in the Hotel. It was rather more relaxed than that experience and I found myself with a group I liked. I still had nagging doubts about it though. There was something missing but I couldn't place it at all. What I was very much aware of was that I couldn't see what, if anything, I would get out of it, yet I still kept an open mind as much as I could. All I knew for sure was that I would be in it for the longer term. I'd been quoted the figure of two years when I started, but that was nothing new to me; short term fixes didn't exist in mental health.

The rest of the week I was pretty much killing time. Again, this was nothing new. I still went along to the Day Service a couple of times. They didn't offer me much but the contact was still vital. Tom had left some time before to go off to an out of hours project. In his stead I saw a quiet and friendly CPN about once a month. The same conversation each month just as it had been over the years but something was better than nothing. I was still labouring under the belief that they were constantly looking to discharge me. The System was still the System; get them in and out as fast as possible. Thus far I had survived the many culls I had witnessed but there was very much a feeling that that fate would be inevitable at some stage. I was also making my monthly pilgrimage to see the shrink just as I had done for years. And then there was Caroline. The benefit was there but it was still very short term. At least it worked though. I clung to the hope that one day, at some stage in the future, that feeling of well being would last for a longer period of time.

But above all else that autumn, I eagerly awaited the post each morning. For once the brown envelope dropping through the letter box would not be one to be feared. As October moved into November nothing happened. The weeks passed in November and still nothing. There was no panic, merely irritation. After all, Adam had said it would probably not happen until the beginning of December. But December came and there was no sign. Worried I phoned him. It was his return call that sent my mood plummeting again. They were refusing to pay me on the grounds that they couldn't read the dates on the paperwork. Then my failure to query it at the time started to haunt me. There was no news on how long it would take to get paid. Yet again the DSS had shafted me. And with that came the question that haunted so many of us, why me?

Over and over it had happened. Why me? It was another difficult Christmas, the first under the Blair administration, as I languished in limbo. With the lowered mood hope disappeared once again. For all the good that had happened in the last few months, my mind was out of control and death seemed the only way out. That, after all, was the way of the mad. And my madness still gripped me in its clenched fist.

Chapter 28

Trickle to Torrent

Caroline was a Buddhist. Since I had been going to see her people had often asked me about a religious, spiritual or faith side to her work. Fortunately her faith and belief rarely impinged on her art. Although underpinned by her belief and study there was little religious content in what she did. When asked she merely described herself as a Healer. There were elements of Reiki, of psychology, of talking, and of love but neither of us could really describe what she did or how it worked. Perhaps what set her apart from the many others I'd met who considered themselves to be professionals was that she gave freely of herself. There had always seemed to be a barrier put up by others. With her it wasn't there. She made the effort to adjust to those she worked with rather than the other way around. Whatever it was she did, it worked for me. Even in the times when I was away from there and the effects had long since worn off, the incident of the leaping dog was still stuck firmly in my mind. That was tangible even if I didn't understand it.

As the last weeks of winter waned in 1998 I had been visiting her for two and a half years. With almost all of those visits there was some relief from the pain and the instilling of a little hope. It usually faded within hours but it trickled in once a month. There was, however, one aspect of her methods that I found disturbing. The only time when her faith came into it was in her firm belief in the idea of reincarnation. The thought terrified me. In the early years I had looked at children with a sense of pity and sadness. I couldn't see the joy in their lives. I was only haunted by the thought that they might grow up like me. It was a pain that no one deserved and children used to display a naivety and innocence that seemed to make them so vulnerable. The idea of reincarnation brought thoughts of childhood and having to go through all this again. Dying was still so central to my world and my thinking. Even with her help going beyond just a few hours, I always felt that one day, even if I got to a moment of critical mass, I would end up as another suicide statistic. That winter any thought of a major and continuous breakthrough still appeared beyond my horizon.

Closer in view than a distant horizon, going to college was having a small impact on my existence. Pioneers as we were it was proving to be a two way, symbiotic experience. Ian learned from us and that was very important. I enjoyed his company and intelligence along with that of Trish his assistant. The content was often limited but he got me thinking, reading, and, that great fear of mine, writing. My struggles and frustrations with the computers continued but slowly it began to come to me. After all my research into Jordan I started to write. Writing free hand initially I completed a lengthy piece over the weeks of the Easter term. Then came the slow, monotonous process of typing up with a single finger. Most importantly though I was pleased with what I had achieved. The old belief that had been so evident in my Cambridge days began to seep back into psyche. Years of grazing in the fallow wilderness of mental illness had taken their toll in my ability to think and write at speed. It was frustrating at times but the build up of confidence outweighed that. And with that confidence what had once seemed just a pipe dream, a return to Cambridge, might just be a possibility at some stage in the future.

Part of the deal with the course was that we would move onto a mainstream course after a year or more and to keep the support. By about March time, with thoughts fixing on returning home, I started to look at options; my musings headed towards doing another A Level. I also started to make enquiries at Cambridge about the long muted PGCE. The danger for me was leaping ahead too fast, particularly when pressurised by those within the System. What I didn't realise was that I was about to make a dramatic breakthrough.

It was mid March when I undertook my monthly pilgrimage to see Caroline. Although things were going okay the visit was just routine, I expected nothing new, just the usual short feeling of well being. That day though it all changed. We went through the talking, the issues, the confrontation and the Reiki. I came away feeling refreshed, enlightened and better. That was normal too. Only this time the feeling stayed with me, and a breech was finally fashioned in the walls of my madness. Perhaps it was a combination of things, of Jordan, of college, of writing, of work with Caroline. Who knows? What I do know is that from that point on, with the obvious exception of my dates, my periods of instability would be almost exclusively reactive. Many of the feelings were still there, as were the voices, but the intensity and frequency was lessened and could usually be put down to events around me rather than the endogenous and unexplained collapses of the past years. With all that, things moved very quickly forward.

There were, however, dangers in this. I still held a deep distrust of those in the System. My fears, shared by many others, were still of abandonment. I had no way of knowing if this change would be but a temporary aberration or a lasting state of affairs. Whilst I was trying to formulate a plan for the future, that plan was dependent on support and careful use of time. After my previous years of experience, I had learned to expect the worst. Any sign of a breakthrough could lead to that abandonment, and, with that, everything could be for naught. If I was to do this I had to do it my way. I could bank on support from Ian, and Caroline, and my old friends in Cambridge. Others I wasn't so sure of. The shrink knew of my work with Caroline and though he didn't understand it, he did not disapprove. I wasn't so sure about the psychotherapist though.

I had always had the impression that she didn't like me going to see Caroline. Maybe she felt it distracted me from the group or that I was dividing my attentions. I had a healthy scepticism for group therapy, a scepticism born out by my previous experience. The nagging doubts that had haunted me since the previous September began to take on a clarity that spring. The people were all nice and I genuinely felt and cared for them but I had always had a feeling that I was in some way different. Some things they talked of just seemed meaningless and irrelevant to me. I'd spent the last seven years with those with severe illness and pain. Much of what I heard, sat on those slightly uncomfortable chairs, appeared milder. There was no doubting their pain but they didn't come across as people with the same understanding as those who inhabited my world. It was in our last session before Easter that it finally came to me. As I sat there painful words from the past illuminated my mind. You're not ill you just have a lot of problems. They were words I had treated with utter disdain both at the time and also in the subsequent years. They were palpably untrue both then and now. Yet as I listened to others talk, the words just seemed so apt. Problems which led to depression. And that was very different to the world of psychosis. I found myself giving in the sessions but not really taking. In one session she seized on that very idea but for naught. The inner mechanisms were mine and would remain mine. I still went in the vague hope that something would come out of it. What that something would be was unknown but in my mind it was worth trying for.

On Good Friday an historic peace deal was signed in the Northern Ireland. The men of violence finally agreed to put away the guns and a form of peace ensued. That Easter there was a difference in my life too. Things were moving. That in itself was alarming at times but after the stagnation in the wilderness a change was welcomed. At the same time there was one area where I was still stuck. My battle with the DSS remained completely unresolved. In fact, despite the good offices of Adam, they had done precisely nothing. They weren't even answering the phone. This hung like a shadow over all that had happened. By May I decided it was time to get help elsewhere and that meant the local Member of Parliament. Having a former cabinet minister as an incumbent had to count for something. It was very early on a cold May morning when I rose for the short walk to the local library to meet him. Outside in the car park a large 4X4 provided shelter for his beshaded security team. I waited in the lobby before the man himself emerged from a door to my right and led me into a small narrow room that I'd never noticed before. I sat and recounted my story. His face betrayed a feeling of surprise at what I'd been through. He took details on some official forms and promised to look into it. I'd never really cared for the man or his beliefs but I was struck by his efficiency and compassion. He was not what I had expected at all. Perhaps it was just another stick with which to beat the new government; that was, after all, the function of the opposition, but he did appear to be genuine and sincere. He wrote to me within a week to tell me he had set the ball in motion. It was the first of many letters from the House of Commons I would receive over the coming months.

It was at the start of the summer term that I began the process of going home in earnest. I made contact with my old tutor in college, the admissions tutor and my old friend Chris. Meetings were arranged with the former pair and Chris invited me to dinner. I spent a very pleasant and productive few days in Cambridge securing references and finding out the lie of the land. I dined in splendour on High Table with Chris followed by the lavish event known as "Combining" complete with vintage port and Madeira and a gilded ram's horn conveying snuff from right to left. The following day we visited the School of Education and the specialist college catering for the teaching of teachers, emerging eventually with the relevant course guides and application forms. There was but one disappointment with the visit. It had always seemed to me that if I were to make such a great step as going back there would be a need to live in college and be as supported as possible. Sadly it proved that my old college could not accommodate PGCE students so I would have to look elsewhere. That said though, I had taken the first step. The next would be to get the application to such a point where it would be very difficult for them to turn me down. There was, however, a whole summer to perfect that though. For now I had the acid test of mid June to contend with.

It proved to be a normal June. For three weeks or so I was intensely ill. Some years later Ian would tell me that he often felt that I would be one of the casualties who would not make it through the year. He learned early that he merely had to look at me to tell my state of mind. Yet through it all I kept going. However badly I was feeling I never missed a day of college or school. It was much harder when I was ill but I had strong sense that I didn't want to let anyone down so I just carried on. In fact it provided a new means of expression. Since leaving school ten years before I had written but one poem and that was when I was in the Hotel. Now as I languished in my private world I started to write again. Through that summer term I wrote prolifically. Some were better than others but they kept coming. I was even challenged with a time limit. James was now heading towards the end of a course at Art College. With his final exhibition looming he decided to tackle the thorny issue of the Archbishop's Palace. What he produced with photography and painting I agreed to try to match with words. Somehow I made the deadline. It was my first step towards really describing such a terrible experience. Pleased though I was with the outcome it did little to ease the pain and fear despite repeated questions from others about whether it had a cathartic effect. The Palace was still the Palace even if much of it had been knocked down. There was no erasing of the scars.

As the long summer holidays began I was beginning to shake off the June slump. The first year of what had been named Open Door had come to a successful conclusion. I was writing again and semi computer literate. A place to study A Level philosophy awaited me in September. School was winding down. A plan was under way to return home, possibly as early as the autumn of 1999. Things were looking good. But I had long since learned not to trust too much in a healthy future. For all that was good there always seemed to be at least an equal measure of bad. I was still waiting for my money. There had for some time been an ominous silence from Rachel. Whilst there had been a great breakthrough near to home across the Irish Sea, the storm clouds were once again gathering in the east. The capital was a few months away from witnessing a new form of bombing campaign. On 12th July France won the World Cup on home soil; England's campaign had been marred by the sending off of David Beckham against Argentina. And, two days after that final, a man was finally arrested and charged with the terrible attacks just up the road of two summers before. Although I had not nor ever would meet him, he was a man who would have a bearing on my story. His name was Michael Stone.

Chapter 29

Legal Recourse

That summer was far from normal for me. The usual sedate pace of the warmer months, punctuated by the evening revelries, was turned to what passed for frenetic in my world. There was simply so much to do. Faxes passed to and fro Cambridge and Kent concocting the wording of the application. Carefully and deliberately I completed the hand written part. Nothing was left to chance. I started to read for Philosophy. Trying to steal a march on time I reread John Mill's *On Liberty* in anticipation. It was a slow and at times painful experience but one that seemed necessary; come September the reading would increase. My reintegration with the old Cambridge crowd continued with an invitation to a dinner in September. It didn't seem like ten years but time was marching inexorably on. So much of that time had been wasted. I had met many extraordinary people but at what price? I could see no benefit to have come from my years of illness. Now there appeared to be a possible escape route but it was daunting prospect. So many what ifs. Yet all I could do was focus on each little step. What had for so long been but a fantasy was now starting to take real shape.

As the pace of life quickened there were constants and there were changes; it was not just me who was moving on. The subtle shifts in our close knit group became more pronounced. People shifted their lives and there relationships. Laura was back from Portsmouth and Jayne would move on to Cambridge that autumn. We still partied but it was not the same; drift, in some cases, became chasm. And all the while I recorded those changes in my new found passion for poetry. One thing that was constant that summer was the stream of letters from the House of Commons. Another was the still deafening silence from the DSS. As the weeks passed and autumn was approaching I started to look for a solicitor to help. After one false start I found one towards the middle of August and an appointment was made in London for the first week of September. In between time I had another birthday and the peace was shattered in the Northern Ireland by the devastating attack at Omagh by a Republican splinter group. The outrage was so great that it proved to be the last such attack. Of course none of us knew that at the time.

Neither did I know that death would be back in my life with alarming frequency over the next three months.

My visit to London that September brought almost immediate dividends. I met a young, clearly able and ambitious lawyer for about an hour. He took copious notes, gave me a card ready to call him at any time, then set to work. It was costing me nothing yet the tax payer paid some price, each and every correspondence adding to the bill. Within a week they had paid me some of the money owed. The hard part would prove to be getting the balance, and, getting my benefit book brought up to date. Correspondence continued.

The success of the visit was quickly tempered by the news that there were too few students to run the course in Philosophy and that I would have to do it essentially alone through Distance Learning. That would be delayed by having to send for the course materials. So I waited and occupied my mind with John Mill to try to get ahead; I would have to wait until the end of October. By this stage my application for Cambridge was honed and ready and it was a question of plunging into the unknown. That step was taken when I first went to visit Jayne in Cambridge.

September 1998 marked the tenth anniversary of our initial foray into the great world of academia give or take a couple of weeks. To celebrate dinner was organised by friends at the old college. My rehabilitation was by then almost complete. I set off armed with a Dinner Jacket, weekend stuff, and the precious application forms. Late in the afternoon I took tea with the Senior Tutor, gave him the forms and took my leave. It was now out of my hands and a question of waiting, but it was a very significant step back towards reality. Dinner of course was splendid, as was the company. After much consumption I headed back to Jayne's and continued the partying for the rest of the weekend. It left me with curiously mixed feelings, a sense of triumph, but one tinged with fear. Could I actually do it?

Not long after my return I heard the tragic news that another friend had committed suicide. A deeply troubled young man whom I'd known for a few years had jumped off a building in the town up the road. He was the fourth of my friends to die by his own hand. As with all the others, it struck me as a release from so much suffering.

A Pillar of Impotence

Within a few short weeks, another would die from a gunshot wound. As I hurtled towards an unfamiliar world I was reminded that my life was still part of that other world, the world of the mad where nothing is ever quite as it seems. Days after the first death I travelled to a new destination; Portsmouth was gone but Nottingham was in my orbit now. Travel was still a constant for me but this trip was overshadowed by the sad news. We had reached the middle of October.

The murky world of Mental Health grew darker on 23rd October. That was the day that Michael Stone was convicted amid somewhat controversial circumstances of two murders and one attempted murder. Within a very short space of time one of the two principal witnesses against him withdrew his evidence. The conviction would subsequently be quashed and a retrial ordered; Stone would be convicted again at that retrial. A crime of such magnitude provoked outrage throughout the country, and, as details of his life published, there was an inevitable backlash. And the target, as I had suspected since the crime was committed, was the mentally ill. He was a man with a history of drug abuse and violence. He also had a diagnosis of Personality Disorder. It was the first time that I had ever heard that devastating and damning phrase used in public. It was a term that held great resonance with me and one that I despised. Now it was a new kind of buzz phrase.

Public fear and disquiet brought a rapid response from government. The effects of that response would impact on far more people than those with the label of Personality Disorder. There seemed to be a loophole in existing legislation, one which essentially meant that someone could only be detained if his or her condition was considered treatable; Michael Stone's condition was considered to be exactly the opposite. To placate public opinion the government proposed a new Mental Health Act. Amid lurid newspaper headlines it was suggested that some people would be locked up indefinitely, potentially for crimes that had never actually taken place. Compulsory Treatment Orders were also suggested.

This reaction, however well meant it was, had a two fold effect on those inhabiting my world. Firstly it massively increased the stigma that existed in society as a whole; those with the throw away label fared even worse than most. Secondly, in an effect that was perhaps more keenly felt by the mad, was a terrible sense of fear. Who would be locked up? Will it be me? Who will decide? These were the unanswered questions on all of our minds. As ever with a government so backed up by spin the announcement was long on headlines and short on substance but that was enough to create a lasting and profound impression on those afflicted.

There was a strange and personal footnote to the Michael Stone case. A few weeks after the conviction the grapevine began to operate. One of the major terrestrial TV channels was planning to film a programme about Stone and was putting out feelers for anyone who had had problems with the Mental Health System, or associated systems such as the DSS who was prepared to talk on camera. I was, of course, a prime candidate for such an interview. Indirectly I was asked if I was prepared to do so. I thought for a long time about what to do, and, as was my wont, took wise counsel. Some felt it was a worthwhile exercise; most did not. The legal advice was to steer clear of anything associated with Michael Stone. I didn't take the risk, and, as far as I'm aware, the programme was never made.

The end of the trial coincided with the long awaited arrival of the package to start my studies. Much to my annoyance, Mill was not covered in the material. Instead I was left with four other texts to read, and to work my way through a particularly fat folder of information designed to teach me the intricacies of the world of Philosophy. Two months late, virtually alone, and with an eight month deadline I set about Descartes, and Hume, and Nagel, and Sartre. My weeks took on a methodical aspect as I slowly worked my way through a mass of material. Most days I went into the college to study the package on my own. Much of the reading I did at home in the late afternoons or early evenings. It just became part of my routine along with school, the group, and the Day Service. And all the while I waited for news. Knowing how I normally reacted to letters that might bring bad news I had a sense of dread with each passing week of the arrival of the post; Cambridge was still out of my hands.

The letter arrived one cold November morning. Surprisingly I opened it immediately. The contents were longer than I had expected. It summoned me to an interview on a Tuesday in early

A Pillar of Impotence

December, the day of the Varsity match. But it wasn't as simple as just an interview. It was also required that I deliver a five minute talk on why History should be taught in schools and some unspecified written exercises. Mystified by the latter the prospect seemed infinitely more frightening than it had appeared. In addition to both those aspects I also had to somehow dig out old school certificates to prove my qualifications in Maths and English; again a worrying prospect as I had absolutely no idea where I would find them. Despite these apparent difficulties I had achieved the first part of what I had set out to do the previous summer. It was now back in my hands

My studies were partially impeded by these requirements but I did manage to get both done in the end. There was one unexpected problem that appeared out of nowhere. The week before the interview the quiet, mild mannered consultant told me he was leaving that Friday. I had always known deep down that it would probably be harder to be passed medically fit to go than to get a place. Now that prospect became harder. I travelled the very familiar rail route to Cambridge the weekend before the interview. Jayne treated me to an excellent couple of days during which there were surprisingly few nerves. It poured with rain that Tuesday morning as I walked nearly two miles to Lensfield Road with no umbrella. Before me awaited a woman whom I knew by name and reputation and another unspecified interviewer who had been identified as a teacher. Drenched, I arrived to find a young woman who appeared to be lost. I assumed she was another candidate; she was in fact the teacher. At the top of the stairs I met the woman I would come to know as Christine who ushered me into a side room. There were four of us there, a woman who was older than me and a man and a woman who were still students. I assumed they were all from Cambridge; I was wrong about all of them.

The writing exercises were deceptively easy, merely requiring us to comment on some text books and to write some prose. When it was over we were all left in a small room to wait our turn to go in. I was the first to be called. The talk went according to plan and was well received. Then came the questions. Some were of history, the bulk were about my health. As had happened in my tribunals time seemed to stop in there but it was a much more comfortable experience. I have no idea how long I was there, but it passed and I emerged to collect my coat from the small room. The other three looked exceedingly nervous and concerned about how long I had been in there. It meant little to me as the concept of time had disappeared. Most importantly though I was out in time for the match. I adjourned to the nearest pub for lunch, a beer or two, and an afternoon of rugby. As far as I could tell it had been a good day despite the rain.

Once again it was time to wait, wait and study. This time the wait was much shorter. The week before Christmas a letter stamped with the University of Cambridge mark arrived. I was alone in the house, alone but for George the cat. With unusual haste I opened it. A place awaited me the following September. There was but one stipulation, to get through an Occupational Health check. That, expected though it was, tempered my mood a little. Nevertheless it was time to celebrate. I spoke to many people that day but nobody came. Alone in the pub that evening my mood crashed; it was what usually happened at that time of year. That morning, I thought I might get through the holiday period okay. I was wrong.

We spent Christmas at Miriam's house. It was an isolating experience as I fought my demons and my way through the dense and almost impenetrable work of Hume. On my return I hoped for a better New Year but it was not to be. Wracked by the flu I attended yet another funeral on New Year's Eve, the third suicide in as many months. Good always seemed to be followed by bad. The flu made it worse with additional hallucinations. Thus I entered the final year of the 90s, the year I would turn thirty, and maybe finally return home. Yet again my fate lay in the hands of others, the people I distrusted most, Doctors.

Chapter 30

Coffee in Gomorrah

Throughout my journey amongst the mad, certain traits seemed to keep popping up; loneliness and isolation were prominent with so many. These traits operated on more than one level. It was almost universal for those who got ill to feel that they were the only ones. This was partially alleviated as they began to filter into the System. Yet there remained the fact that each individual's experience was completely unique to his or herself. Some had the skill of empathy, others did not. We listened to each other and understood in a way that was known only to the mad but it was impossible to know exactly how each experience felt to others. Most of those whom I had met were single people, with or without children. The comment that "if I could only get a girlfriend I would be okay" was one I heard so often from young men. From women more often than not it was a case of avoidance of a partner. Unusually I fitted more into the latter category than the former. Those who lived alone, and there were a large number of them, had physical isolation to deal with along with the loneliness of detachment. With me it was often too dangerous to be alone; needing someone there, anyone, had been the backbone of my DLA claim. It had been very rare indeed that I had been left alone for more than a few hours for most of the decade.

I was still waiting for the bulk of the money at the start of the last year of the twentieth century. I was determined more than anything else to do one thing when it arrived, and that was to go on holiday. Due to the lack of payment I had missed out on a trip to Amsterdam with friends the previous summer. The plan was to rectify that when the giro arrived. I wanted to see Van Gogh. When that desire would be realised was unknown. What I did know was that I'd probably have to do it on my own. I wanted to see the demons of a genius in a museum but I also intended to face my own.

Time took on an enigmatic character that winter. After recovering from the flu I got back to the grind of Philosophy. The dirge of Hume gave way to the delights of Sartre, then the complexities of Nagel. The work seemed to go at an enormously slow pace, yet each passing page and day drew me closer to the time of reckoning in

June. The fabric of time warped and twisted through two opposite poles, slow yet fast, long yet short. Anticipation and fear speeded the days up but the work itself slowed them down. January sped into February but the pages seemed to disappear at a snail's pace.

Whilst the work became part of my new found routine, a routine in which progress could be measured, in the rest of my life nothing changed much. I was still waiting for the brown envelope which would bring good news, and there was no news of when that would be. More worrying though was trying to meet the stipulations laid down by Cambridge. I saw a locum consultant in January. Yes, he assured me, he would write the report for Occupational Health. In February he was gone, replaced by another of his ilk. No report had been written. The promise was made again.

It was a kind of limbo for me, one that was different from that of the past but equally frustrating. The plan was in place, and so far, had worked to perfection. All the years of them trying to move me out of the System had been for naught; what I had done I had done largely on my own. The talk was always of moving on for all of us; the old adage of getting people off the books as soon as possible, a belief held by almost everyone I'd met who had had the misfortune of entering the System, still held sway. Yet the one thing I needed to make it possible was lacking. No one was prepared to commit to writing a single report, one that held my life in the balance. As with the money, no time scale was evident. I had no idea if I would see the same person in March as I had seen in February, nor indeed in April or May. There was a time limit to all of this; by late summer it would be too late. Great progress had been made in the last year yet I still refused to believe anything until it actually happened; bitter experience had taught me neither to believe nor trust. And so the waiting went on.

When change finally happened it came like a set of dominoes cast into motion by some unseen being. It was March. Once again genocide was at work in the East and the name Kosovo was all over our TV screens and newspapers. NATO intervention was imminent, a case of when not if. I was still in Kent working away on the last remnants of the vast tome I'd been sent the previous October. In the second week of the month I finished it. All the work was done and the texts read. An entire A Level syllabus complete in four and a half months; completed entirely alone. Simultaneously an unusually fat brown envelope dropped through the letter box. Inside were a letter and a giro. The former explained that I could not cash the latter as the amount was too much and that it would have to be banked. The amount included compensation and legal costs to be paid by me to the London solicitor who had helped me. All told the incompetence of the chairman of the tribunal had cost the tax payer nearly £1000. I was now about £5000 richer.

The following day I banked the money, walked into a local travel agents and saw a familiar face.

"How can I help you?" she said.
"I want to book a few days in Amsterdam." She got out some books and made some calls.
"What's going on in Amsterdam?"
"Nothing, I'm going to see Van Gogh."
"That sounds good." A few minutes later it was booked. My journey to slay my ghosts was set for the last week of the month. It would be almost exactly ten years to the week since my previous visit to that curious city with its mix of sin, culture, tolerance, and hostility. With me would come my baggage and my fears. It was time to face the tribulations of isolation and loneliness.

The NATO air campaign that would last for seventy eight days, destroy the infrastructure of a country but apparently little else, and bring with it an influx of refugees who would for ever change the make up of my part of Kent, was but a few days old when I flew from the London City Airport to Schipol. After a very early start and having fought my fears of getting lost, I made it to my small hotel about two hundred yards south of Dam Square by mid afternoon. Unloaded, showered and briefly rested, I emerged into the sun lit city and headed off in search of coffee. Three joints of Thai grass later I left for a wander with the words of so many of my friends ringing in my ears, "go to the Grasshopper." More than anything else though I needed beer; smoking without alcohol, especially weed was a sure thing to bring on the paranoia for me.

My travels were accompanied by the sights, sounds, and the people of the city. The families, the individuals, the pimps, the prostitutes, the dealers, the tourists. Each represented another face of the place, and each was calculated and evaluated in my drug addled mind. Some were safe and some were hostile. Of equal input were the dangers of speeding bicycles and trams. Eventually as I walked along a narrow street I saw a sign saying "Grasshopper." Like so many of the other coffee shops I had passed on my way it appeared to be a small underground establishment; it was only later that I realised it covered the whole building and this was just part of bigger whole. Entering slowly I was delighted to see that they served beer. I sat at the bar and ordered a small beer from a very attractive blonde girl. It was only after I had been there a few minutes that I realised the danger. A giant of a man from the former Dutch colonies was towering above the other customers. As he paced back and forth he downed spirits at an alarming rate. Each time he opened his mouth he spat aggression at all those around him. Get out. What the fuck are you doing here? Why did you come? The mind, laced with paranoia, swept into overdrive. There were no voices; just sheer terror. Looking around it was obvious that all those there felt the same. Yet that was no help. I have to get out. Finishing my beer I slipped as surreptitiously as I could from my stool and went for the door. In absolute fear I realised he was following me out. Had I been in England I would at least have had the advantage of understanding the language. Here my fear was compounded by a lack of comprehension. He's going to kill me. Get out. As I glimpsed the last remnants of the sunlight in the street I set off to my right. He went left. Badly shaken and questioning my foolishness for ever coming to Holland, I ambled along in a haze of paranoia.

I found myself in an old, dark, wooden bar.

"What can I get you?" said the young fair haired man.

"A large beer please." It duly arrived. Exhausted from my 5 o'clock start I nearly passed out at the bar.

"You look very tired, are you sure you don't want coffee instead?" I marvelled at his immaculate English and that wonderful accent.

"No thanks, beer will do me. After three I'll be fine." Three pints later I was indeed more awake, much to his surprise. I left looking for food. My mind was still in turmoil, and, in the end, I had to buy some Nepalese hash to calm me down from the Thai grass. It had been a most curious day and I was deeply contemplative that night as I anticipated Van Gogh.

A Pillar of Impotence

As a child I missed many lessons due to the weight of music that made up my days. Art was one of those subjects that was deemed dispensable. The result was an untainted and uneducated view on what is known as art. The great advantage of this was that I came with an open mind, one that could be swayed by my own beliefs, observations, likes, desires, and opinions. I could appreciate art for myself not from the view of critics, teachers, or practitioners of the brush, pencil, paper, or canvas. It was with this in my mind that I set out nervously for the Van Gogh museum. With the help of a friendly native I ventured onto a tram and arrived at my destination at lunch time. Much to my annoyance I found that the museum was shut for renovations. With my hopes rapidly disappearing I was saved by the small print. Part of the collection was on display at the Rijksmuseum just up the road. Taking lunch on the way I entered the vast building and followed the signs for Van Gogh.

The exhibition was set out over three rooms with directions given to follow a particular path. Never being one overly enamoured by convention I decided to progress at my own behest. It was rapidly clear that here was something astonishing to behold. I'd seen the pictures in books but to be so close took me into another world. The *Sunflowers* was there in its magnificence. I moved from picture to picture, pausing often to watch those around me. I wondered what it meant to them and their levels of appreciation but it was impossible to tell. Slowly I meandered back and forth. Having completed the first two rooms, I slipped into the third through the wrong door. Nothing could have prepared me for that room, the one with the paintings from the asylum days and beyond. There before me was the menacing desolation of *The Plough and the Harrow*. It changed the whole mood of the rooms, darkening and deepening them. I had no need to look at the guide plaques for I was back in my own world, the one I had inhabited for the past decade. And here was a man who had been dead for one hundred and nine years bringing that world to a surreal life. Time took on its familiar distortions as I observed the works of a true genius telling my life and that of so many of those I'd met along the way. He simply portrayed madness in its greying yet brilliant light.

Those around me seemed to float out of the room and indeed my very existence. Mesmerised and astonished I moved around buffeted by the imagery of madness. I was transfixed by *The Raising of*

Lazarus for half an hour as I stared into the face of the artist in the paleness of the oils. How could someone do this? This is my life. He has captured its essence. My mind raced as it marvelled at those priceless objects. I thought of my own feeble attempts to explain my world but nothing compared to this. The room itself exuded pain and anguish. It haunted me but I had no desire to run, simply one to soak it up. As I became exhausted by the experience I glanced back at my watch. I had been in that one room for two hours. That was as much as I could cope with but I left determined to return, my life enriched by those few hours.

Over the course of the remainder of that day and those that followed I ate, drank, smoked, read, visited, and wrote in my own time. Unencumbered by the will of others I moved about under my own will. There was joy, sadness, exhilaration, fear, despair, happiness, and paranoia. I visited Anne Frank's house. Finding a large queue outside, I took up residence on a small bench outside and contemplated the extraordinary significance of that otherwise unremarkable building, one just like the others in the street. There seemed to be more to be had from the experience than going in with so many others. Van Gogh was done again. And all the time I lived with my loneliness, fears, and voices. It was a fight in that strange and occasionally hostile wilderness, a wilderness in which I knew no one and met few. Tired or lively, drunk or sober, hungry or full, stoned or straight I took each day as it came, slowly winning the battle that had been so virulent in my mind for so long.

On the last night of my visit I ate, drank, and smoked, just as I had done on each night. Yet sleep would not come. Too much going on. The hours drifted by slowly. As it started to get light I took an early and brief breakfast then set out into the sleeping city alone with my thoughts. Little stirred out there. Over the next two hours I watched that sleeping city come to life as the sun rose higher in the sky. It promised to be a glorious spring day. With my flight scheduled for early afternoon I returned to the hotel to pack and return my key. The quiet and polite dignity I had come appreciate of so many of the Dutch was in evidence as I said my goodbyes and headed for the Grasshopper for the last time. I was very calm as I walked up to the station after.

As was my custom, the result of fear, I arrived very early and purchased my ticket. With time to spare I walked on through the station and found a whole new world. Amid glorious sunshine I sat down and watched the water taxis ply their trade to and from the quay. As the people came and went I was alone in my world. I talked to Rachel but there was no response. Quiet, my mind was quiet. The calm became a peace unknown for years. She was there but she was silent and less haunting. As I sat there I finally started to let her go. For a brief few moments there was no turmoil and she was no longer my nemesis. It was an astonishing moment, brief in the scheme of time, but one that would have a lasting impact on me.

The journey back was not without its train hitches but by late on a Friday afternoon in the spring of 1999, I was through customs and on to the Docklands Light Railway. The politeness of so many of the Dutch was replaced by coarseness of the British working man returning home and gearing up for a Friday night drinking session. I had returned to the United Kingdom and reality. The coming months held their fears and joys. As I sat on the train that mattered little. Every emotion known had touched my being over those few brief days. I had survived my demons and laid to rest some ghosts; I was changed and one more significant step had been taken. It was sunny here too.

Chapter 31

Circular History

There was one question asked of me that had dominated my years of illness from the very beginning: Was it pressure of Cambridge that caused it? It was a question I'd fielded from a wide variety of people, some in the know and others not. The answer was always the same, an emphatic no, the pressure only came afterwards. In fact the question was not as simple as it seemed at first sight. There was the direct part which was one of causation, high pressure working environment leads to breakdown. The indirect implication was known to fewer perhaps more astute questioners, who put on that pressure for you to succeed? What troubled me was that no one appeared to accept the answer. It was me who challenged my self to succeed. I went to Cambridge the first time for me, not for anyone else. I had not been sent away as I child, I had chosen to go. Maybe the legacy of the violence of that childhood played a part; that was the part I had neither chosen nor expected. The man I knew simply as god had described my expectations as "ridiculous" and taken it to be evidence of a disordered personality; so had his predecessors. I still held the firm belief that I had an illness, one that would have been evident to them had they bothered to talk to anyone who knew me before; with the exception of Rachel they had singularly failed to do that. The quiet, mild mannered shrink I had visited for several years raised questions and fears for my return to Cambridge. Would it be too much for me? Would it bring back damaging old memories? Maybe, maybe not. I wanted to return home and do it for me. Yes there was the need to try to carve out a late career, and to prove the doubters wrong, but going home was the big motivator. They didn't seem to get that either.

With the exception of the almost ill fated trip to Chartres three years before, all my musical trips had been at Easter since the age of fourteen. Amsterdam had been a rarity along with Jordan in that it was a non working visit. Yet that spring I found myself in a position that was both familiar and daunting; another countdown had started. Eleven years previously I had returned from Seville to do the exams that would ultimately take me back to Cambridge. Three years after that Barcelona had been my destination before my final and devastating descent into madness. Somehow I had held on long enough to put myself in my present position. A second return was almost imminent, possibly. Before then though was the matter of testing myself again. The future was not entirely dependent on that test but it mattered to me, and that was what had always mattered most. Expectation was rife, but only in my mind.

The countdown began just after Easter when revision started in earnest. Using my traditional method I slowly whittled down the notes from the pack to more manageable sections. At the same time I reread all four of the texts. The dates arrived not long after I started to revise. There was an immediate problem; one was at precisely the wrong time in June when the illness was likely to be at its worst. There was nothing I could do about it though. Two and a half months was all I had left, but I envisaged that they would be relatively free months. With the exception of trying to get the medical report written, nothing else was on the horizon.

That all changed early in May. A large brown envelope dropped through the letter box. Knowing who it was from it lay unopened for a few days. Thinking foolishly that my problems with the DSS were behind me it was most unexpected. When I did open it I found a form called IB50. Its purpose was to justify myself yet again. A date was given for its return and it was emblazoned with the warning that if it was not returned any benefit could be stopped. I knew that the next step would be to go for another of the infamous medical tests at Canterbury. Memories of my previous visit flooded back causing alarm and delaying my revision. I was accustomed to fearing the worst and this raised the spectre of having to get a job at some stage before my planned return to Cambridge. A job and the A Level. Too much. The plan was unravelling before it came to fruition. There was, as ever, no explanation as to why I had been singled out, but that was what I had come to expect from them. No peace.

Whilst I worked I continued with all the other things in my life. School went on each week and proved to be a useful blessing when an edict came from Cambridge requiring me to do a full time week in a Primary school in either July or September. I was still attending the Day Service once a week or so. With Tom long gone and my temporary assignment with a CPN ended I now had to work with an older woman who seemed to hold some position of authority. Often

I wondered how on earth she had got to that position. She was model of bad practice, always late, cancelling appointments without telling me, and asking why I hadn't told her I would not be coming when I had done precisely that. She irritated me. Within a couple of weeks of receiving the form she suggested there was no problem getting a job and doing the A Level. I simply walked out after an eight year stint.

As I had done for the last eighteen months or so, I travelled to Ashford for the group on a Tuesday night. This was also becoming something of an annoyance at times with the mundane regularly being the norm rather than the exception. Often I came out feeling far worse than when I had gone in but I persisted. Caroline was still Caroline though.

As the weeks of May rushed by, the war went on with little in the way of progress apparent to an expectant public. No one it seemed had expected it to take this long. I was making progress though with Philosophy. Unfortunately the same could not be said about getting through the requirements. In May I saw a different locum again. The promise was made but not honoured; still I knew not whether I would be going or not. Maybe June would be different. Time was ticking away on all fronts. The trial was barely two weeks away. So was illness and fear lived on.

Those two weeks passed rapidly, and, as expected, illness came. Two days after the crucial date I found myself in a sparsely populated sports hall in Dover on a gloriously sunny day. Three hours to face and quell the voices and thoughts. The paradox of confidence and dread filling my otherwise blank mind I fought through the first few minutes. Nothing went down on paper as all I had learned of Philosophy stubbornly refused to come to me. Panic began to set in. Then from nowhere it came back to me. Ink flowed through an ancient pen not used for so long, flowing if a little shaky, years of medication having severely limited my ability to put words down legibly. When the three hours were up I was done, confident yet shocked at how I'd stood up to the test.

A week later I returned to that same sports hall, my mind slightly clearer than it had been. This time my only companions were the seagulls padding around and screeching above me. The allotted time went more quickly that day but I got it all done. With a tremendous sense of relief I left and went straight to the pub. It had taken me seven months but I had achieved what I'd set out to do. Now once again it was time to wait for the deliberations of others, others who were unseen. That would be the big test but I left with belief and expectation intact.

With one more hurdle crossed June turned to July. That brought my week in school. This, like so much before it, would be another test. The burning question was whether I would have the stamina to do it. Fighting an accumulation of exhaustion I made it through an enjoyable five days there. Again there was a mixed effect on me; on the one hand I proved I could do it but on the other it added a little to the trepidation of having to do it full time. A week was long enough but a fifteen week second term that was planned for the following January seemed a most daunting prospect. Only time would tell that though and there was still one more obstacle to over come first.

He was an American, another unknown. It was bright July afternoon when I walked into the Day Service to meet this month's locum. Time had almost run out. He had to commit to writing the report. The initial pleasantries observed, I had to directly challenge him. Much to my surprise he agreed to write it. Hope started to grow. Then it happened.

"Well," he said, "I've been looking at your notes and it would appear I have two choices about diagnosis, Personality Disorder or Psychotic Depression."
"If you put down either of those things I'll never be allowed to work with children again." My mind raced off again. The Personality Disorder was expected but the admission of a psychotic illness had never been made before. True though I believed it to be it would never help my cause. Depression was the only way forward much as I loathed that word. What really got to me though was that someone, somewhere had accepted but never bothered to tell me or treat it. I'd been in the System eight years and finally the truth was out but one that would completely wreck my plan.

After much wrangling he accepted my position and acquiesced to my request. The label I had always hated became my salvation.

He must have written the report shortly thereafter because within a week of so a letter came from Cambridge. It confirmed that I had been medically cleared. I was going home. Relief poured out of me. What had once been a pipe dream, a fantasy, was barely two months away from becoming a reality. There remained one more summer to try to enjoy despite the rather lengthy reading list that had arrived.

Four years had passed since that epic summer of 1995; things had changed. Some had moved on and were seen only occasionally. Others were still living in the small seaside town in Kent with the little pub at the bottom of the hill but our relationships were more strained now. The old crew was scattered and more divided than at any time in the 90s. Overall it was a much quieter town now. There were parties but they were more spaced out and sometimes fraught that summer. Still waiting for a response from the DSS I enjoyed what I could as time drifted on to my departure date.

One thing that didn't change was me getting ill early in August. Shifts in my illness had been pronounced over the last couple of years but it remained in a rather more latent form. Cambridge was coming but I was still vulnerable. For all the progress, deep in the back of mind was the belief that one day suicide would claim me. Pills were the preferred option and although they had been less frequent and often less intense, thoughts of suicide lurked almost everyday. I was also grimly aware that in many respects life was about to get much tougher. I was used to dealing with the mad world, now I had to face the real one as well.

With but a few weeks to go and in dreadful despair, the brown envelope dropped through the letter box. It was the day of the eclipse. Leaving it in the house I wandered slowly down to the beach to witness the event. An eerie silence descended as the sky darkened; even the waves seemed to lie still. An unusual calm came over my mind blotting out the ravages of an unquietened space. As the sun reappeared I moved off back up the hill determined to open the letter now. The contents surprised me. No they weren't going to take away my benefit or make me get a job. It also said that there was no longer any need to send in sick notes every six months. It was a supreme irony, for eight years I had had to get the notes and pass them on. Now, but a few weeks from returning to some form of normality they were no longer required. A rare victory.

A Pillar of Impotence

The days of August took on a new speed as I waited for the results and for my thirtieth birthday. Not long after I had left the Hotel the Evil Pixie had rather disdainfully commented that there were only "five years to thirty." That time had elapsed and I was on the threshold of getting out of the world of the mad. At the time I doubt either of us had any belief that that would happen. She would never see my return and she remained mourned by few. I had almost done it and with but a modicum of help from them. My nerves though grew with passing of the days.

Results days always seem to be trumpeted by the press and government alike. Standards are rising was usually the mantra. It was warm in Kent when that day arrived. I phoned but had no luck; grades could not be given out over the phone. The slip of paper was at the Dover branch and could be accessed if I came over. Having recently mourned the demise of the battered old yellow VW, I climbed into the somewhat newer if less conspicuous car and drove up the coast. In the office I was handed a small envelope. Stepping outside into the sunshine I opened it quickly. Stunned was the next feeling. Two grades below what I had wanted. Again. Terrible memories of illness and breakdown swept over me. I looked in sheer disbelief. History had repeated itself in more than one way that summer. Failure. That was my perception. The shock was not just within me, no one could understand it just as they hadn't done all those years before. The feelings lasted for days. A subsequent appeal was less than fruitful and I was left to grudgingly accept that it had served its purpose. I had failed there but nothing could deter me from my ultimate goal.

With my thoughts still tinged with a sense of failure I turned thirty on a sunny August Bank Holiday Monday. That was the day we traditionally held the Day of Decadence party, an idea resurrected from the old Cambridge life in the rather different surroundings of a sleepy seaside town. It was generally a good day but degenerated as the cracks and fissures of our muddled lives became more evident later. Another day of consumption and another day closer to home. I had about three weeks to go.

There were still things to do in those last few days. Most of the paperwork mountain of loans, references, and identification had been completed. There remained such things as clothes, equipment, the dentist, the optician, and a myriad of details. It was a time of anticipation and anxiety in almost equal measure. There was also a certain amount of reflection. It was hard to believe that I had come so far, from the coldness of coma and death to the light of the future. I often got the impression that most people around me assumed that was the end of the line; go back and get on with my life. I was more pragmatic and circumspect. It was going to be very tough but getting a job at the end would be tougher. But I kept my thoughts to myself, pondering them in the rare quiet moments of a still warm early autumn.

The only remnant of my former routine left in September was my Tuesday nights over in Ashford with the group. Annoying though it had been at times I had kept going for two years. I couldn't really place what if anything I had got out of it but I hoped I'd had some impact, however small, on the lives of the members. Indeed the therapist had once observed, maybe very shrewdly that perhaps I should do more taking and less giving. On the Tuesday before I was due in Cambridge, I had to go to the see the dentist prior to the group. I emerged with two new fillings, and a very numb mouth from two injections. Still unable to feel my mouth and barely able to speak, I arrived for my final session, a time for goodbyes.

"I'm sorry but I'm not sure I can speak very much tonight as I've just had two injections at the dentist's."

"Maybe that means you just don't want to speak," came the response from the therapist. Bollocks. That just about summed up my views on therapy. I'd been in it in one form or another for most of the last decade yet I still had little idea of what it actually meant. Even at the last they were coming out with the same old bullshit. The goodbyes were made at the end but I had few regrets about leaving. I have only ever seen two of the members since. One I passed by in the street near my parent's house. The other, a fellow student of mine, I've seen twice. He left about a month after I did; the words "not ill just a lot of problems" had had an impact on him too.

I made arrangements to go to Cambridge a day early. Saturday was the day I would return, ready to register on Sunday afternoon. There was one last Friday night to get through before that though. I expected just another relatively quiet night with a few friends as I made the short journey down to the pub at the bottom of the hill. I bought a beer and headed for the back room. It was full; they had come from miles around to see me off. For one night only our differences and fractures were set aside for a mighty party. Like that day in the summer of '95, the one on which I had turned twenty six, they had come to see me.

When the pub closed we headed for the beach loaded with take outs on a clear and warm night. The party went on long into the night and early next morning. As we sat there, a strikingly violent thunderstorm whipped down the Channel. Lightning forked into the sea as we watched in perfect safety. The powerful symbolism of that night often entered into my reflections in the following years. We stayed dry and marvelled at the ferocity of nature, just a fleeting presence for one last night.

It was later than I had planned when I awoke on a Saturday morning in September 1999. Before me lay the task off packing, and driving a once familiar route to the north. My parents were rather emotional as I bade them farewell but immensely proud. I had been ill since 16th June 1990, nine years and three months. I was still ill but alive and more in control than I had been in all those years. As I drove down the slip road onto the motorway I reflected on what I had left behind. More than anything else that was the biggest change in my life. There was something left behind this time. But time had moved on. I felt some emotion and sadness as I drove but what lay ahead was greater. Finally, almost literally back from the dead, I was going home.

Chapter 32

Et Resurrexit

I have a certificate dated 1st August 2000. It bears the signature of the Right Honourable David Blunkett, Member of Parliament, the then Secretary of State for Education and awards me Qualified Teacher Status. My return from Cambridge to the small seaside town on the Kent coast was a triumphant affair. Emotionally and mentally I was on top of the world. I had achieved what I had set out to do long before I had actually returned home. As it transpired this was a major shock to many, particularly in the medical profession. Although none of them had said it at the time, few believed I would return and survive the rigours of teacher training. And rigours they were.

It had been an extraordinary year. Mighty highs and great depths accompanied the sheer volume of work to be done and hours put in. Christine had asked me at my interview how I felt I would deal with the inevitable disasters that went with the course. My response had been that they could not possibly be as bad as those I had already suffered. I was both right and wrong on that point. The problems in themselves were not insurmountable but when they made me ill then I faced an almost impossible task. I had two major and intense periods of illness during that year; both almost broke me. They were compounded by the fact that very few people there knew of my illness. Christine was an immense support to me and to others. Those around me were also hugely helpful although they laboured more or less in the dark.

Perhaps the most moving moment of all was right at the end when we all went round to Christine's for a garden party. Part the way through she pulled me one side, away from prying ears. In a quiet, secluded corner as the heat of a summer's day receded she told me two things that will always stick with me. She revealed that when she had first met me she had wanted to accept me on the spot. Due to the exceptional circumstances she had felt that she needed to consult with her colleagues; all of them advised her against taking me on. Her other comment really surprised me. She had always made it abundantly clear to all of us that she considered those who went through the training and then did not go into teaching were wasting her time and resources. My case was different. She didn't care whether I went into teaching or not but what really mattered was the great triumph of getting the qualification. Triumph or not there was one problem that faced me as that summer progressed, and that was that I did not have a job for September. There were a few others in the same position, history being one of the most competitive markets for teachers, but at least they had had interviews. Not one single school in the whole nine months of the course had even shown me the courtesy of wanting to meet me. All my applications had been greeted by either a rejection letter or a deafening silence. There didn't seem to be a market for damaged, tainted, or otherwise risky goods.

In July that didn't matter very much to me. In a rare victory over bureaucracy the IB50 I had filled in with great fear the previous summer still held true; my benefit was restored at its original level. Although I had spent almost all the money I had and gone into debt to the Student Loans Company to the tune of nearly £4000, I was still receiving my DLA until the end of August. The scene was set for a memorable summer.

The cracks and breakdowns of relationships seemed to matter less that year. Wiser possibly, and definitely more tolerant than before, life proved to be good in the warm months of summer. I had more places to go now rather than being occasionally stuck when people weren't around. More calls to make and another world in which to escape when I felt like it. Those I met along the way shared my good fortune and welcomed me back. There were new things to talk about, no longer just the mad guy who had to dance with the real truth. Respect was due to teachers, albeit unemployed ones, more than there was to a nutter. I was more socially acceptable than I had been before; the eccentric now had rightful place in society and was, at least theoretically, contributing to that society.

My mood remained buoyant on the whole. Even early August was easier to deal with; my dates were still my dates but the intensity was diminished. Part of me even began to think that there was a possibility of maybe coming off medication. That would take time and I would have to be realistic but it was an idea I could not even conceptualise but a few months before. Although I was jobless once again I had faith and belief that that would only be a matter of time. In the interim Ian suggested that it might be an idea to try to get a Learning Support job at the college and come and work with him. That was an idea that appealed but was initially thwarted by a waiting list.

In late August my income was drastically reduced by the loss of my DLA. I had felt I didn't really need it anymore but Heather insisted that we reapply anyway just in case. The application was rejected outright on the evidence of my GP in Cambridge who had last seen me very well. Although it made life more difficult all remained well in my mind.

After my birthday summer gave way to what would prove to be a very wet autumn. With autumn came the start of the job season for teachers. There was an initial trickle in September, then more. Like the rains of autumn the market would crescendo into a river in late October and November. The floods around Kent proved the background to renewed hope of work. A little breakthrough occurred in October when I finally received news that the college wanted to interview me in November for a possible start on Open Door in January. A small beginning, a platform on which to build, and some more money coming in.

I was interviewed on 8th November and offered the job an hour after I left the campus. It had even been suggested that if I were to work less than sixteen hours per weeks I might be able to retain some of my benefits and maintain a small income during the unpaid holidays. One of the few sops the DSS had to those who were ill was the Therapeutic Earnings Scheme. It had helped one old friend and now seemed perfect for me. Life was looking up. Sadly that hope would last a mere twelve days.

On 20th November 2000 I suffered a devastating relapse and went into complete mental melt down. The following morning a large envelope lay on the mat after a night of non existent sleep. It bore the unmistakable hand writing of Rachel. I'd not heard from her in over two years despite her promises to meet up on her return to the country. Inside was a pile of old notes I'd lent her years before, notes which I had been requesting back ever since the possibility of the PGCE had come into being. There was also a post card. It told me that I had indeed been right all along about them. It also announced that she was about to get married and move abroad in the New Year. Without Heather and the timely intervention of Beka taking me to Bristol I would not have survived the week.

I had not been in the System for over a year. Now, apart from those in the mad world, I had no one. In despair I went to see my old GP. She took a brief look at me, talked for a while, then sent a fax to the Mental Health Team requesting that I be seen and assessed immediately. That fax was ignored. There was no call. As each subsequent day passed I waited in vain. And with those days the voices howled, sleep betrayed me, and my mind continued to break apart. Death was once again the only answer.

Two weeks later I was forced to go back to my GP. She was furious. A second fax was sent, the phone rang and an appointment was made for a couple of days hence. It was a cold, damp, and overcast day in December when my father drove me to an unknown destination to re-acquaint myself with the people I call shrinks. Before me sat a frighteningly young and attractive junior doctor with a foreign accent. The questions were all so familiar. She made me uneasy because it was clear that I knew far more than she did. After an hour or so came the answer: a change of medication. The little blue and white capsules had been my lifeline to sleep for seven years were to be mine no more. She proposed that I reduce, then come off them in a week. In their stead would be another pill that would help me sleep and be more effective. Remembering the terrible withdrawal effects I'd had from my previous medication, I resolved to come off them more slowly. Then she asked me to let my parents look after them for me. No way was I going to let that happen; they were my lifeline to sleep but also my means of death. After that she and the consultant asked to speak to my father alone. More memories of the past flooded back. A follow up meeting was arranged for the New Year and that was that. Back to where we had started and there didn't seem to be any difference in the way the System operated from before. Once again I was alone with my demons.

Whilst all this was going on, there were also the details of getting ready for the job and getting the required approval of the DSS to deal with. Both organisations appeared to thrive on reams of paper. At that stage I could barely even read. Somehow with the help of

Heather the former details were sorted before Christmas. Approval was still some way off with time running out.

Christmas, always one of the most difficult times of my illness, proved to be one of the worst ever. Things actually got infinitely more complex over that period. I didn't think it could get much worse but it did. Barely clinging to life I staggered into 2001, a time I thought would hold great promise but which now seemed chronically empty.

I had but days to go until I was due to start my first ever job post university. Still there was no word from the DSS. Alone I had to go in there. Eventually they found the letter from the GP suggesting it was a good idea to work. It also said she didn't think I was well enough to do it at the moment. Against this advice I chose to go ahead. The bureaucrat told me that was okay. The consequences of that conversation would not become clear for eight months; unwittingly I was now on another collision course with my old nemesis.

Two days after that meeting I drove to work for the first time. Over the next two and a half months I worked three afternoons per week. I coped only because I was back amongst my people, those I knew best from my life with the mad.

My follow up with the new shrink took place at the end of January. I was still on the old pills, trying to wean myself off them. Nothing had changed. She told me there was no point in being on such a low dose as it was ineffective. I didn't give shit about her opinion. When I did start the new ones there was no effect. Still no sleep and utter despair. Unbeknownst to me they would have an effect but not the desired one.

It started very slowly, almost imperceptibly. It had always struck me over the years that despite my weakened state it was extremely rare for me get physical illnesses. From the moment I went on the new pills that changed. At first it was the occasional cold, diarrhoea, then the ear infections. As time passed they became more and more frequent. After a while my GP had serious concerns about my hearing and referred me to a consultant; but that would take months.

There appeared to be no obvious reason for these physical ailments. I just had to put up with them.

There was no change in my mental health though. The young shrink had seemed quite uninterested when I saw her in January. The follow up was left until March. A few days before I was due to see her that March I received two rather unexpected calls on the same day. Two schools, both wanting to interview me for a teaching job. At last things were beginning to happen and my mood rose. They both wanted to see me on the same day, the day I was due to see the shrink. After making arrangements to travel and fit both interviews in on consecutive days I called the Mental Health Team to change the appointment. I was met by an answer phone. Leaving a message I explained the situation and asked to reschedule my appointment. They never got back to me. It would be four months before I had contact with them again, time in which they had no idea whether I was alive or dead. At my worst they still didn't seem to care.

Both interviews ended in failure but there were positives. The feedback was good but it was not enough to stem the slump after. Those two days in March set the trend for the next few months. As the weather warmed in the spring the phone regularly rang with offers from schools and colleges. It seemed that once I had got one job and someone was prepared to take a risk others followed. Each time I had a call my mood rose, then, with each new failure it fell again. It helped a little but I was painfully aware that time was finite. The well that was so deep in the spring and early summer would run dry by about July.

Time ticked by, April to May, then May to June. June that terrible month for me. It was now eleven years since I had become ill. Now, with my mental health in turmoil, my physical health continued to worsen. My visits to the GP became increasingly regular but no treatment helped. The concerns about my hearing were more urgent now. The other problems had become an every day occurrence. Still there was no word from the Mental Health Team. By mid July, convinced that it was the new medication causing it, I walked into the building that had become so familiar to me over the years and made an appointment. The young foreign girl had finished her placement and a man was now in her place. As it transpired he too was about to finish his time there.

It was a warm day in late July, not unlike the one almost exactly ten years before when I had first seen the professionals that I walked in there. I was furious at being left for dead. Taking an unusually aggressive stance I let rip about what the medication seemed to be doing to me and my feelings at their incompetence. Rather taken aback the young Dutchman before me said he had never heard of such side effects but I could, if I wanted to, come off them. That was a relief but the other issues were left unresolved. Why had I not been seen? He couldn't answer that but he would have to check with his secretary. Looking unnerved by the whole meeting, he told me that he was leaving at the end of the week but I could see his replacement the following week to look at what to take instead of the medication that was apparently causing all the problems. I will forever remember his parting shot:

"I think you'll like my replacement, she's very experienced." As I left my thought was simple, experienced at what?

That July the jobs well had, as expected, run dry. There had been such a positive response from most of schools. I had had a very close run at one but it fell through at the last minute. But the bottom line as I faced a long summer holiday was that I was still only partially employed in what I had hoped was just a temporary position. At the end of August I would face two months with no other money coming in but my benefit. The words "you're depressed because you haven't got a job" were beginning to run true as well as my illness. Into this chaos stepped the DSS. Another IB50 arrived and the prospect of a medical, and all that that entailed, began to loom again. I had tried for nearly two years to get work but had failed. It was yet another factor bearing down on an over worked mind; the dream was unravelling. And still my illness was tearing me to pieces. Maybe it was time to die.

It was another day of turmoil as I drove to the hospital. I had no expectations but that I was about to meet yet another shrink who didn't know what she was talking about and wouldn't believe a word I said. The years had brought extreme cynicism and the hope that had existed a year before had all but faded to extinction. I sat alone in the small stifling waiting room; another day at the office. After a short while the coded door opened and out stepped a woman in her thirties. She introduced herself in a mild Scottish accent and led me upstairs to a small office. Nothing in her demeanour suggested she would be any different to her predecessors. We sat down and the ritual started. It was then that I realised she was different. She came straight to the point. That was different. She had read about me and taken a clear interest. Most of all she spoke my language. She spoke as one person to another, not the clear professional and nutter approach of so many in her profession. But most importantly she listened. It took her ten minutes to completely shock me.

"What do you think you have?" I'd never been asked that before.

"I accept that there is a major depressive element to my illness but I have always believed that I have a psychotic illness."

"Do you think those two are mutually exclusive?"

"No, of course not, but no one has ever listened to me."

She was listening though. It was unprecedented in my experience. We talked some more. She completely dismissed any notion of a Personality Disorder. As she put it "when I first came across the concept of Personality Disorder in my training I realised that I must have had at least six different ones at various stages of my life." Like me she considered it complete bollocks. Then came a cataclysmic statement.

"I don't think anything you have been told is true. It sounds to me as if you have a Mood Disorder. Have you ever thought about going on a mood stabiliser?"

"Do you mean something like Lithium?"

"No, I was thinking along the lines of Risperidone." Alarm bells rang out. Both a Mood Disorder and the drug Risperidone were very familiar terms. Many years before one of my friends had been misdiagnosed with Schizophrenia. It had later transpired that he had a Mood Disorder. Amongst other drugs he had been prescribed Risperidone and it had gone a long way to helping him get his life back. I'd not heard of its use as a mood stabiliser but I had had heard nothing but good about it and its track record for stopping voices was well known.

I was now in completely uncharted territory. In a small room I was with someone who spoke my language, was listening to me, completely challenging the deliberations of others, and she was offering me a choice. It was an option, but there were others. After about forty minutes, with time running out the choice would become mine. She was clearly shocked at what I had told her of my past and my treatment. As I prepared to leave there was one final thing to take care of.

"Do you have access to the Internet?"
"Yes."
"I'm going to write down the names of three drugs which are options. Go home and look them up."
"I don't need to look them up I need to talk to my people."
"What do you mean? Are you part of some sort of group?"
"I'm going to talk to the people who take them. They'll tell me what I need to know." This seemed to surprise her. But it had been a day of surprises. With an appointment set for the following week I left.

Walking across the car park I ran into an old friend.

"How did it go?" she said.
"Put it this way, I've finally found someone I can do business with."

Throughout August we met every week or two; it was what she called "aggressively" treating my suspected, if as yet unnamed, Mood Disorder. Meeting her was an astonishing breakthrough for me but I was still very ill. I talked to many people about what the options were as well as looking on the Net. The latter told me very little as Risperidone was only rarely used as a mood stabiliser. Neither I nor anyone else had heard of it being used for this purpose.

Each time we met we talked in the same meaningful way. I came off the other anti depressant and almost immediately most of the side effects ceased. The ear problems continued for a while but eventually went away. It was only many months later that I discovered that that particular medication could have a profound effect on the immune system; I was one of the unfortunate few affected by this. She refused to put me back on the old blue and white capsules on the grounds that they were unsafe. Even with the dark connotations of suicide I was able to be completely honest with her. We talked too of potential side effects of Risperidone and the other options. Yet again this was new to me.

Whilst all this was going on the storm clouds continued to gather and thicken. The cause of my relapse had been removed from my world in May. Now it was coming back. The DSS confirmed that I would indeed have to face the dreaded medical at Canterbury. I had thought that life couldn't get any worse but it seemed to be by the day. An old saying from the bible kept popping into my head, "fat bulls of Basan close me in on every side." Basan, the place that had been at the start of my first recovery; recovery seemed such a long time ago now.

My decision to try Risperidone was taken quite early. In fact I had dismissed the other two options on the very first day. I was troubled by but one thing. Barely a year before I had been contemplating coming off medication completely, now I was faced with the prospect of having to take not one but two different types. One night in August I sat in the pub at the bottom of the hill with James and talked my way through my dilemma. His advice was quite simple:

"If you think you need it, try it."

At my next meeting I agreed to try it. She told me to wait a few weeks to see if the new anti depressant would have an effect. I accepted this and waited a couple of weeks. In the event it had no effect.

Three days before I turned thirty two, a final devastating hammer blow was delivered by the DSS. Another brown envelope arrived. Inside was the news that they had assessed my earnings and were cutting my benefit. The estimate was wildly wrong. An enquiry revealed that they had never actually processed my Therapeutic Earnings properly; neither had they granted permission to work. Effectively they were claiming that I was working illegally. The news came the week I received my final pay for two months. That was for one week's work. My benefit was slashed to £40 per week; I would have to live on that for the next nine weeks and there was nothing I could do that was legal to get any more.

It was probably a Tuesday the next time I saw her. The anti depressant had done nothing. It was time for the final gamble. Very close to death I agreed to take Risperidone on the proviso that if it did nothing after three months I would come off it. I had no expectations of it, just another attempt to treat what had proved over the years to be stubbornly untreatable. Armed with a prescription with the instructions to take one milligram at night I left and headed to the hospital pharmacy. That night I took two different pills for the first time.

The effect was instantaneous. It was also almost miraculous. Heather noticed it the following night after but one pill. Over the following week my life totally changed. All the symptoms vanished. A calm I had never known in all my life descended on my mind. What had been dark was replaced by a brilliant light. The blurred became clear. There were no voices, neither was there any desire to die. My mind was still and rational. The abyss into which I had been thrown disappeared; there had been neither walls nor floor in my tunnel, just me, floating in darkness. The subterranean lift exploded through the surface, settled and remained there. The lights were on and finally, after eleven years of pain, I was alive. Alive, and glad to be alive.

Epilogue

It was never my intention to write beyond my return to Cambridge; circumstances changed that. The impact that Risperidone had on my life was instant, dramatic, and far reaching. Yet it is almost impossible to describe to anyone not on it. It gave me back my life but it was a new life. I was no longer the person I had been before Rachel but I had been through years of therapy and was now eleven years older. A great deal of reflection followed which led to a most unexpected and surprising conclusion: the advent of Risperidone made it so clear to me that I have probably had a Mood Disorder most or all of my life; there are even those who have suggested that it was inherited. All my life but it had lain hidden, inert, inactive until that terrible day in June 1990.

Not long after I went on it I had a brief conversation with my mother. She told me that I had talked of having chronic mood swings even when I was at school. Looking back on what had always seemed very happy times I recognised this; what really surprised me though was that I had ever said that to her. Now I had a new perspective on life as well as a desire to live. And along with that, an unusual calm that I'd never known before. Everything became so much easier to deal with.

Despite this wonderful sensation I was very mindful that it was not all over and I would for ever be vulnerable to a return to illness. It was still very early days as I took the first steps into a new life, a life I was aware I still had to work at.

The reflections were not just about the past. There were two things that were now abundantly clear to me. Firstly I had an enormous sense of triumph and self justification. Secondly came the realisation that something had gone catastrophically wrong in the way in which my case had been handled; and that led to a lot of questions to which, personally, the answers were irrelevant, but were very relevant to others.

Back in the days of the Hotel, that last chance of salvation, god had made two comments that had always stayed with me. "I'm not going to give you a diagnosis as you might think that you can find a better shrink who will be able to help you." The notes proved the lie of that statement. "I don't think you will ever find a medication that will help you." Translation, you don't have an illness. The open, listening Scottish Doctor and Risperidone completely destroyed his statements to me. He was wrong. I had spent four months with him; she identified what she thought was the problem within about ten minutes, treated it "aggressively" as she put it, and that treatment had worked in a most dramatic way.

I had never changed my story since the day I first entered that stifling Victorian building in the early summer of 1991. In 1993 the Dutch counsellor had come up with the concept of the subterranean lift which so exactly described my condition and a form of a Mood Disorder. I had always felt I had an illness, an opinion shared by so many of those who had known me before, but no one wanted to talk to them. I found out many years after that Miriam had been there the day they took me to the Palace. They treated her with contempt yet she knew me. No one was interested.

It was in 1996 that the Chartres incident occurred, possibly the most disturbing and frightening experience of the whole time period. The mild mannered shrink listened, questioned, and then did nothing. Risperidone was on the market then. It is of course pure conjecture what might have happened had it been prescribed then. Sometimes I wonder how I would have been had I discovered the drug earlier; how much of an impact the subsequent work with Caroline and Ian would have had will never be known but it is an interesting question. What I do know is that although Risperidone is prescribed to me as mood stabiliser, it has had an astonishing effect in obliterating the voices. I have rarely heard voices since then. Each time I do, I know that if I take three milligrams instead of the usual one, they stop.

When I met the Scottish Doctor I had spent nearly ten years in what we call the System. She was visibly shocked by my story. But what surprised her most was that mine was not an isolated case. I have met many extraordinary people over the years who have had similar experiences. There was so little trust and faith in those who are trained professionals. To many they are the enemy. The pervading sense of hopelessness that litters the lives of such people is matched by their feeling that they have been failed. To give up lends credence to that lack of hope.

In my case perhaps that greatest failure is that no one challenged decisions that were made without any input from me. Choices were always loaded, explanations never given. Once I had that devastating diagnosis of Personality Disorder I was finished, written off, consigned to the dustbin. I had questioned from the start. It seemed logical that if I didn't respond to an idea or treatment, either or both had to be wrong. The answer was not that it was me; it was that they were wrong. When a different answer came my life changed.

I consider myself enormously lucky to have found a solution as simple as taking one pill. Most of us who have what those in the business call Enduring Mental Health Problems are not that lucky. It may seem odd to anyone reading this for me to consider myself lucky. After all, it took a decade of almost unrelenting hell to find a solution. Sometimes I think I should be very angry about what happened to me. At times I have been but I'm not now. Yet one of the more unusual properties of Risperidone is that it takes away the need to ask the question why. Quite simply the answer doesn't matter. It is a property others on the drug have noticed as well. What does matter though is asking the question for those who are not as fortunate as me.

My time in the System was not wasted. I spent those years talking to, and, more importantly, listening to some of the bravest and toughest people one could ever meet. The fact that many face life and death all day every day brings a certain wisdom unknown to those who have not felt such trauma. It was these people who made it worthwhile.

Of the hundreds I have met over the years I have no idea how many are still alive. I personally lost nine to suicide; that's only the official figure, others too having died by their own hand but not recorded as such. But suicide is not the only killer amongst the mad. Physical complications, eating disorders, side effects, drugs and alcohol, and other illnesses all reap their toll. It is one of the great tragedies that so many conditions are misdiagnosed because a patient has a history of mental illness. And many of those die far too young. Death comes in many guises. When we fail people the unpalatable truth is that the consequences can be fatal. This is not just confined to those who are ill but also to those thankfully rare but publicly trumpeted cases of homicide. Each death is a tragedy.

Unfortunately the issue of high levels of mortality is compounded by other factors. Perhaps the most driving of these is poverty. Whilst the Department of Health sets targets to lower suicide rates the Department for Work and Pensions sets targets to get people off Benefits and into work. The two don't mix when it comes to mental health. At least one of the suicides in my life was as a direct result of the actions of the latter department and its previous incarnations. I was hounded by them every step of the way. It took me another year after I found Risperidone to finally get away from them. Nothing was made easy for me. The demands to justify one's existence by the DWP heap untold misery on those afflicted with this blight. I'm not aware if figures are compiled of deaths and hospital admissions caused by the apparent assumption that nearly everyone is on the take. Sadly our cause is not helped by the fraudsters.

For all the pressure there is to work, what is rarely talked about outside of my world is just how tough it is to get a job with a label of mental illness. It took me eight months to pass a medical to take up my PGCE place and even then it was against the better judgement of many experts both medical and educational. When I finally had an opportunity to get off Benefits with a second part time job it took over two months to get through that medical. At Cambridge I had a ten year gap in my CV, one that for so many schools was an insurmountable difficulty. I never made it in teaching; after two years of unemployment no one wanted to know. It was not until June 2003 that I was able to secure my first full time job; by then I was nearly thirty four years old.

After my third stay in Cambridge I learned what depression was. Depressed because I was unemployed and had no money. Depression is not the same as me being ill but the former makes me vulnerable to the latter. It's a terrible condition to have.

Perhaps the greatest irony of my story was that when I finally got off Benefits and into work it was a job within the System that did it for me. Since then I have worked in both the statutory and the voluntary sectors. It was an eye opener working for what had always been the enemy. Most work extremely hard, sometimes with mixed results, others not so. What is clear is that work loads are often ludicrous and expectations high. Too often there are too few staff managing too many cases. Money has always been an issue; resources are stretched. These are the issues that recur so often at meetings.

But it is people who make a system work, however flawed that system may be. It has long been a system whereby need, the word we always hear from professionals, is decided by those professionals with little input from the people who matter. We can't even agree on a name for them: clients; tenants; service users; patients. In the parlance of so many we are nutters, psychos, loonies. Who are we? What are we? We are people with difficult and complex needs. Historically we have never trusted others to assess those needs. There have been signs of improvement but it is often limited to the lucky few. To an extent the System remains a lottery based on where one lives or who one's GP is. To get a good professional too often depends on that. We need more and better quality people. And that means recruitment and training as well as resources.

Mental illness is becoming much more recognised now but there is a long way to go. There remains great stigma, fear based on ignorance. What people don't like to recognise though is that it can happen to anyone; no one is safe whatever one's background. I led a very privileged life and had the best part of a decade fighting what often seemed a losing battle; and that battle was a very lonely one at times. Maybe that is the most important lesson of my story.

Therapy in all its guises is becoming more openly talked of but is still not as acceptable as it should be. The old asylums have gone, the Palace is now a housing estate, and we are picking up the pieces of the catastrophe that was Care in the Community. The long heralded and highly disputed new Mental Health Act came into force in 2008. It was not as the government wanted but we now have Compulsory Treatment Order; in the first year applications for CTOs amounted to ten times the Department of Health's estimate. Times are changing and we can but hope that those changes will be for the better. But we have a great distance to cover before those in need learn to trust again; there are simply too many out there with experiences similar to mine. Perhaps it is time to look again at what they like to call Personality Disorder; it is a damning verdict on people who have needs that are not being met. I could so easily have laboured under that label for the rest of my life when in fact the solution was quite simple. How many others are there out there who have been misdiagnosed? How many have been consigned to the psychiatric dustbin? The answer may never be known.

Despite the pain and anguish of the 1990s I have few regrets. It was a time in which I have met some of the most courageous people I could ever hope to live with. I learned all the time and continue to do so. Each of us has a story to tell and lessons to pass on. I consider it a privilege to do what I do, to be let into so many lives. I probably face a life time of taking medication but that is just an accepted part of my life. I have an illness, but it is one that for the most part is under control. But it remains a work in progress. There is very little malice in me although there are those that I fear I will never forgive. That's the work that remains to be done on my part.

It took me almost exactly three years to write and recount my story. When I reread it I find much of it I have forgotten. For years this story in all its detail revolved around my mind. It doesn't any more so maybe it has served its purpose. Those three years were anything but easy at times. People asked me if I kept notes or a diary. I didn't, all of this is from memory. Some of them thought I would give up after a while; that was never an option for me. It had to be done.

Shortly before I started to write I went to a party in London with my old friends from Cambridge. They had seen and misunderstood the start, now they saw me well again. Early in what proved to be a memorable night I talked to a woman I'd not seen for many years. She said something that really surprised me: "You must be so strong." Odd was my first thought. But later I reflected on what she had said. Like so many of us I had to have had strength, the strength to survive. Yet I had been powerless in the face of my illness and the treatment meted out to me over the years. It had a certain resonance. Strong yet powerless. A Pillar of Impotence.

Lightning Source UK Ltd.
Milton Keynes UK
172445UK00001B/11/P